DOCTORS AT WAR

DOCTORS

THE CLANDESTINE BATTLE AGAINST

ELLEN HAMPTON

LOUISIANA STATE
UNIVERSITY PRESS

AT WAR

THE NAZI OCCUPATION OF FRANCE

FOREWORD BY PATRICE DEBRÉ

BATON ROUGE

Published with the assistance of the V. Ray Cardozier Fund

Published by Louisiana State University Press
lsupress.org

Manufactured in the United States of America
First printing

Designer: Michell A. Neustrom
Typeface: Sentinel
Printer and binder: Sheridan Books, Inc.

Cover photograph: Red Cross workers on boulevard Saint Michel evacuating
a wounded person as the uprising begins in August 1944.
Copyright © Agence LAPI/LAPI/Roger-Viollet.

Library of Congress Cataloging-in-Publication Data

Names: Hampton, Ellen, author. | Debré, P. (Patrice), writer of foreword.
Title: Doctors at war : the clandestine battle against the Nazi occupation of France /
    Ellen Hampton, foreword by Patrice Debré.
Other titles: Clandestine battle against the Nazi occupation of France
Description: Baton Rouge : Louisiana State University Press, 2023. | Includes
    bibliographical references and index.
Identifiers: LCCN 2022032178 (print) | LCCN 2022032179 (ebook) |
    ISBN 978-0-8071-7873-7 (cloth) | ISBN 978-0-8071-7944-4 (pdf) |
    ISBN 978-0-8071-7943-7 (epub)
Subjects: LCSH: World War, 1939–1945—Underground movements—France. |
    Physicians—France—Biography. | World War, 1939–1945—Medical Care—France. |
    France—History—German occupation, 1940–1945.
Classification: LCC D802.F8 H35 2023 (print) | LCC D802.F8 (ebook) | DDC
    940.53/440922—dc23/eng/20220706
LC record available at https://lccn.loc.gov/2022032178
LC ebook record available at https://lccn.loc.gov/2022032179

This book is dedicated to those who know when it's the right time to break the rules.

CONTENTS

ILLUSTRATIONS

FIGURES

MAPS

FOREWORD

Resistance Past and Present

I am writing from Madères, the Loire Valley estate of my grandfather, renowned pediatrician Robert Debré, where a paved court ends in a small structure of brick and stone, topped with a slate roof. This building, which abuts the imposing main house, was erected by Count Ostrowski, a Polish military officer and refugee from the Russian annexation of Poland in the early nineteenth century. Finding safe haven here in the Touraine region, he built the stable to close the courtyard, where yellowing leaves pile up in autumn from the neighboring woods and insistent weeds emerge around the paving stones in spring.

It would seem a quiet place, tranquility broken only by a game or the step of a horse, if it were not for the odd holes driven into the stone wall. As children we would stick our fingers in the holes, but they are not natural to the stone. They are bullet holes, and by their side, etched in stone by a dagger, is a swastika, only partly erased by time. These are the traces left by German officers who occupied the house in 1944, using it as a regional Kommandantur. The details of the requisition are spelled out in an official document we keep on a chimney mantel.

These are present reminders of a harrowing past. It was to this house, long before it was requisitioned, that Robert Debré fled when the Gestapo came to arrest him. He was in his Paris office, in the middle of a medical consultation, when the men in trench coats and fedoras came to take him. Slipping into a clandestine life, sought for arrest by the German police, he continued to direct resistance work against the Occupation. Yet when he was stripped of his right to teach and practice in public hospitals because of his Jewish ancestry, it was not only the will of the Nazi regime, but also that of Vichy France. When they tried to impose a yellow star on him, he refused to wear it, out of either courage or pride.

These episodes and many others are found in this well-documented book, along with the names of both great and less well-known actors of French medicine, those who made history as part of the medical resistance, and those who made medical history after the war. We meet these heroes in secret networks fighting against the occupier, organizing sabotage, acting with courage and at the risk of their lives. We learn the multiple levels of active resistance, from fake identity papers to false diagnoses of dangerous epidemics. They fought against German oppression and against the dire effects of anti-Jewish laws. Ellen Hampton writes with detailed focus to bring to life the tension and drama of this medical resistance. While this is not her first World War II history, it is perhaps her particular talent to evoke the perilous atmosphere of the time.

My grandfather is not the only hero included, far from it, but it is to him that I owe this foreword to the book. And so we return to Madères. My grandfather spoke rarely of the Occupation; it became submerged in the horror of the concentration camps, which he visited in the aftermath and was seized by the terror and degradation experienced there. He wrote about it in his autobiography, and he no doubt considered that was enough. But then Madères brought forth a new and original source of documentation. Robert Debré kept, in the early period of the Occupation, a daily journal, which lay hidden in a locked cabinet, unknown and unseen until recently. This handwritten journal offered his personal views and impressions of the calamity unfolding around him with an immediacy that enlivens this narrative. In fact one of the great qualities of this book is its delivery, as history, of what it was like for the men and women of that terrible time, the mix of glory and shame, the silence of some and the courage of many, the compromises, the insanity of men. As the writer remarks, the actuality of the past is told in bullet holes and the ink written day by day.

But it seems to me that it is also important to understand these historical events because they reverberate into the present. They allow us to look into the depths, beyond the anecdotes, and offer perspective on this life today. The fight against human rights abuses is not in the past. Is academic freedom not swept aside in numerous nations today? The medical profession continues to be undermined by false prophets. People have died for giving vaccines. Ideologies continue to punish and stigmatize oppressed minorities for their origin, religion, or sexuality. Some reject science and fear knowledge. Amplified by the power and spread of social media networks, fake news, alternative facts, propaganda, lies, and disinformation—as well as partisan politics and anathemas—have in effect massively invaded the public spirit, relegating science at times to a subordinate role. It was also against such oppression by a dominant ideology that the medical resistance was fighting in World War II.

Confined for a time at Madères because of COVID-19, as my grandfather was because of the Nazis, I could not help but wonder if humankind is destined to live through such very sad epidemics, whether biological or ideological. Lacking sufficient power to prevent them, it seems to me important to know the history—such as this book delivers—to better reflect on threats we face today.

—Patrice Debré

Madères, France

ACKNOWLEDGMENTS

Heartfelt thanks go out to the many wonderful people who helped bring this book into being. *Doctors at War* grew from the seeds of a film documentary project proposed by the American Hospital of Paris. Hospital governors John F. Crawford and David T. McGovern had brought the Hospital's early history through the First World War to the screen in *The American in Paris,* and wanted to follow up with a film on its history in World War II. The COVID-19 pandemic put that project on hold. At the same time, my research on the medical community in Paris during the Nazi Occupation revealed a larger story, full of fascinating characters, perilous situations, courageous actions, and difficult choices. Despite the enormous historiography of WWII in both English and French, the doctors' story had not been told. Thus my first thanks go to John and David (we so miss him) and the team at the American Hospital, especially Jérôme Deana, Agnès Touchet-Chazal, and Véronique Cottat. Jennifer L. Rodgers, who led the WWII film research, also played a role in pushing me to look further afield.

Dr. Patrice Debré, whose fine foreword opens the book, provided access to the extraordinary element of his grandfather's wartime journal. I am very grateful to him and to his wife, Marianne Debré, who took the time to explain references and relationships, the key bases for contextualizing the sometimes brief phrases in the journal. Dr. Florence Prochiantz, widow of Dr. Alec Prochiantz, also was an important source, especially for the Morvan region, and generously provided photographs of her husband for publication. Other medical interpretation (what is a *pince de Kocher*??) was given by my dear friends and neighbors Dr. Frédéric Goyet and Dr. Florence de Ruyter-Goyet. Dr. Lorraine Colin, granddaughter of Elisabeth de La Bourdonnaye (as she is called in the book), was a great help in bringing Elisabeth's story to life. Also in the Morvan, Noëlle Renault and René Marin provided solid assistance.

The Nazi Occupation and its terrible persecution of Jews is deeply documented at the Centre de Documentation Juive Contemporaine of the Mémorial de la Shoah in Paris. The assistance there of documentalists Aurore Blais and Anne Huaulme was vital to this project. Professor Laura Hobson-Faure, chair of modern Jewish Studies at the Université de la Panthéon-Sorbonne-Paris, provided a very valuable close read of the manuscript as well as unwavering support throughout the research process. At the Bibliothèque de l'Académie Nationale de Médecine, chief curator Jérôme van Wijland also offered great assistance in finding pertinent material. Thanks are due to Gabrielle Perissi, assistant director of collections at the Mémorial de l'Internement et de la Déportation at Compiègne, and to Dr. Sanders Marble, senior historian at the US Army Office of Medical History, for his help with the US Army's medical organization in France.

I am particularly grateful to Dr. Rand Dotson, editor-in-chief of LSU Press. He offered steady support and enthusiasm for telling the story in a manner accessible not just to scholars but also to general readers. If only specialists in history understand the past, then we are indeed doomed to repeat it. The team at LSU Press has done a wonderful job of shepherding the manuscript to final form. I also would like to thank the anonymous peer reviewer whose comments on the first draft of the manuscript made this a much better book.

Friends and family are always the first to listen to ideas and offer suggestions, and I am very lucky to count among friends Susan L. Sachs, Laurie Kassman, Kathryn English, Laurence Chatel de Brancion, and Fabienne Duvigneau. I am happy to have gotten advice and counsel from Sylvie Zaidman, director of the Musée de la Libération–Musée du Général Leclerc–Musée Jean Moulin, and from historian and author Michèle Cointet. Both my sons, Julien and Austin Urraca, read the manuscript and made helpful suggestions, and my husband, Claude Urraca, provided tremendous support in both the writing and the editing process. I couldn't have done it without him.

DOCTORS AT WAR

INTRODUCTION

I f it were as simple as good vs. evil, the stories would have been quickly told. But the Nazi Occupation of France, from June 1940 to January 1945, was a complex sea of ambiguity, in which innocence could turn to guilt, or right become wrong, in the blink of an eye. Arguments continue today over what was done, or left undone, in that shadow-bound period. Did obeying the Germans mean betraying France? Was loyalty to the subservient Vichy government treason, or patriotism? Many of the French loved Marshal Philippe Pétain for his service in the Great War, but flinched at his handshake with Adolf Hitler in 1940. The writer Jean-Paul Sartre, who stayed in Paris through the Occupation, wrote about it at the end: "Evil was everywhere, every choice was a bad one, and nevertheless we had to choose and accept responsibility. Every heartbeat involved us in a guilt which horrified us."[1]

Doctors stood at the center of this moral labyrinth, sworn to help and not to harm, balancing social authority and professional integrity against economic survival, weighing political beliefs against obdurate power. For some, the choice was made for them: most Jewish doctors were blocked from practicing in the earliest stages of the Occupation. For others, negotiating the maelstrom was guided by personal conviction. Some dove headfirst into organized resistance, some helped out when the occasion arose, and others, a notorious few, worked feverishly to promote the antisemitic, right-wing policies of the new French government, named after the spa town of Vichy, where it made its headquarters.

Antisemitism did not arrive with the Nazis, but had been simmering since the 1930s in the form of growing pressure against immigrants in the professional classes, particularly in medicine. Refugees from the authoritarian and fascist rise in Eastern Europe had sought shelter in France, but even if they completed French medical studies and received a diploma, the government took measures to block them from practicing. In August 1940, on the heels of the surrender, the Vichy government declared that no one whose father was not French could practice medicine in France. The supporters of these measures did not conceal that their targets were Jews. Two months later, the Vichy government issued the first "Statuts de Juifs" law, which, among other restrictions, excluded Jews from teaching.[2] Jewish doctors, even those whose parents and grandparents were French, could no longer do their teaching rounds in hospitals. This was followed less than a year later by a drastic ceiling cap on the number of French Jewish doctors allowed to practice. While these measures targeted Jews in particular, doctors across all ethnic and religious lines had to choose whether to cooperate with such a government or to try to thwart its antisemitic programs and Nazi alliances. The risks were enormous. Treating an injured Resistance agent and not reporting it to the police, as required by law, could bring arrest, imprisonment, execution. Declaring a patient's tuberculosis damage too severe for him to go work in a German factory, if the diagnosis was slightly exaggerated, was an act of resistance. For the Vichy government, these medical acts were considered as helping the "terrorists." There was no middle ground of neutrality, even in medicine.

Those who took strong stands on either end of the spectrum often left traces, either in postwar prosecutions, or certification as Resistance agents, or in published memoirs. Surprisingly, in the tidal wave of histories written about WWII and the Occupation, the story of doctors has been largely overlooked. Individually, their resistance stories are dramatic, heroic, and inspiring, beginning with the German invasion of France in May 1940 and continuing through, for some, years of imprisonment in Nazi concentration camps. This book brings together the stories of a dozen doctors who chose resistance, as well as a few who thrived on hatred. On both ends of the spectrum, they are necessarily a small sample of a much larger, and difficult to measure, group of doctors whose stories remain untold. French historians have noted the names of some three hundred doctors who were deported to concentration camps, most for resistance activity. A Paris Medical School monument honors nearly one thousand doctors killed by acts of war between 1939 and 1945, a figure that includes those who served in the armed forces. These men and women represent a fraction of the 28,000 doctors licensed to practice in France in 1940, in a population of 41 million (in 2019 there were 226,000 doctors for a population of 65 million, five times more doctors per patient than there were then).[3]

Who were the doctor-resistants? Most of them were French, some were immigrants or children of immigrants, one was American. Most of them were men, as women doctors were a tiny minority in the 1940s. Dr. Robert Debré was the son of the chief rabbi of Neuilly-sur-Seine, a posh suburb of Paris that also was home to the American Hospital of Paris. Dr. Louis Pasteur Vallery-Radot was the grandson of the great scientist. Dr. Robert Merle d'Aubigné was the son of the Protestant pastor of Neuilly-sur-Seine. Dr. Thérèse Bertrand-Fontaine was the first woman physician to lead a department in a Paris hospital. Other doctors had been held as prisoners of war after the French surrender, and some were students finishing their medical school studies.

In March 1942, Debré, Pasteur Vallery-Radot, and a small band of fellow doctors organized a clandestine Resistance Health Service, aimed at treating injured Resistance fighters and fallen Allied aviators, as well as stockpiling medical supplies and creating false identity papers. They were a disparate group politically and culturally, but together, they were of one mind: the Nazi Occupation must not be allowed to succeed. They would do whatever they could to bring it down. And as doctors, they were particularly well placed to help the Resistance. They had *laissez-passer* documents allowing them to circulate after curfew, they had widespread contacts across all levels of society, and they had medical expertise and social authority. If a doctor said the man in that hospital bed had typhus, not even the German police would come for a closer look.

They brought hospitals into action, creating laboratories of false medical certificates, aimed at keeping prisoners out of camps and deportees off of trains. In the basement of the venerable Institut Pasteur, they stockpiled medications for use by Resistance members, whose increasing activities put them ever more at risk. They helped Allied airmen, sometimes injured bailing out of damaged aircraft, and hid them with escape-line networks on their way to safety out of Occupied France. Then in September 1943, the British and Americans, running undercover help to the Resistance from England and Switzerland, asked them to organize with other medical groups into a central Resistance Medical Committee, to be led by Dr. Pasteur Vallery-

Radot. The Allies would provide funds and material for their medical resistance work, if they would agree to join forces for the singular goal of liberation. As in any French profession, the spread of political tendencies was wide. For example, a leftist doctor referred to the Resistance Health Service as "the Jockey Club" of the Resistance, a witty nod to the social status of its members.[4] But left, right, and center, the doctors managed to set aside their ideologies in order to concentrate on bringing freedom to France.

Danger surrounded their every effort, not only from government authorities or the German occupier, but from their own colleagues. Hardline antisemitic practitioners, vocal since the 1930s and spurred on by Vichy, wanted to reduce, if not eliminate, Jews in medicine. Among them was Dr. Louis-Ferdinand Destouches, better known by his literary pen name Céline. Another was Dr. George Montandon, a doctor and anthropologist, who responded in 1940 to criticism of his ethnoracial theories that he was not following Hitler's ideas, Hitler was following his.[5]

Historians have tended to separate Jewish deportation from Resistance deportation in the larger context of WWII. The tragic fate of deported Jews has become Holocaust history, while the Resistance is its own field of study. After 1942, Jews were sent to death camps, while Resistance agents were imprisoned in labor camps, whose dreadful conditions led to the deaths of tens of thousands. The cruel difference between the types of camps was often one of immediate murder in the gas chamber or slow murder in the frozen fields. Yet of 86,000 French deported for Resistance activity, an estimated 60 percent returned, most of them physically wounded, all of them emotionally and psychologically damaged. But they returned, in far greater numbers than the 5 percent of Jewish deportees who came home to France.[6]

Dr. Charles Richet was among the returnees, a survivor of fifteen months at Buchenwald. He had mounted a campaign against the strict food rationing imposed by Vichy, warning in 1943 that 10 million French were in a condition of "slow famine," and 2 million of them were threatened with starvation. "The Krauts are starving the French population!" he shouted in the midst of his medical lectures.[7] Upon his return, Richet dedicated himself to working on the pathology of deportation and its medical effects. Three other doctors who started one of the largest resistance networks, Vengeance, also were arrested and deported, worked in concentration camp clinics, and managed to survive. Dr. Sumner Jackson, an American who stayed in France despite the Occupation, was arrested in May 1944 and sent to the Neuengamme labor camp. He worked in the camp clinic, helping fellow internees as best he could under reprehensible conditions. He did not return. Nor did Dr. André Cain, a prominent Jewish gastroenterologist, sent with his wife to the gas chamber at Auschwitz-Birkenau in May 1944.

I began researching the doctors' stories as part of a project on the history of the American Hospital of Paris during WWII. Then came the COVID-19 pandemic, and suddenly, doctors were in the news everywhere, and so were the conflicts that often arise between government and medicine. There was a distinct echo forward as governments across the globe turned to doctors and public health specialists for ways to manage the crisis, and a divide soon emerged between those who spoke for citizens' interests and those who spoke for political or economic interests. Health and politics have often had polarizing relations; what is good for one is not necessarily good for the other, and it is particularly in times of disaster and difficulty that the conflict becomes most evident. In the 1940s, doctors in France were faced with a political crisis that spilled over into health issues; in 2020, doctors all over the world engaged with a health crisis that took on political aspects. Historians will assess pandemic responses in due time. This book takes the doctors of the 1940s into the examining room. The choices they made saved lives in ways they never imagined when they began studying medicine; the actions they took were both an expression of their character and a consolidation of their identity. In these choices and acts, taken in a brief precarious moment in time, they renewed vows of an eternal prescription: *Primum non nocere.*

1

THE SHOCKING COLLAPSE

War fell upon France suddenly, and at the same time seemed as though it had been weighing on the horizon since Adolf Hitler was named chancellor of Germany in 1933. For those who had fought the first round, from 1914 to 1918, there was a strong sense of déjà vu. The peace concluded at Versailles in 1919 appeared to have been little more than an opportunity for Germany to raise and re-arm a new generation of soldiers. From that terrible war, the lessons written in blood and etched in stone in every French village were not only about artillery and tactics. The armies learned that medical services needed to be close to the fighting, with field hospitals and ambulance squads set up in every region, and teams of doctors and nurses embedded in the combat forces. It was not just a question of saving lives; it was also aimed at instilling confidence in soldiers, that if they were wounded, they would not be left to die in the field.

The German invasion of Poland on September 1, 1939, brought the responding French and British declarations of war against Germany on September 3. Mobilization of men in France had begun the night before: as of midnight on September 2, the Franco-German border was closed and some 5 million young men, of a total population of 41 million, were called up to serve. Among them were nineteen thousand doctors, dispatched to various army units and military hospitals, with many of the WWI veteran doctors assigned to command positions.[1] Dr. Robert Debré, a prominent fifty-six-year-old pediatrician, was given the rank of lieutenant colonel and dispatched to the Health Ministry. Dr. Gaston Nora was made captain and sent to a military hospital at Versailles, and Dr. André Cain became commandant at another military hospital. In the previous war, they had been young medics treating the devastating wounds of heavy artillery and poison gas. Now they were behind the front, but not far from the nightmares it still provoked.

A younger generation of doctors, some barely out of medical school, signed up as well. Alec Prochiantz, twenty-five, and Paul Milliez, twenty-seven, became medics. Robert Merle d'Aubigné, a thirty-nine-year-old orthopedic surgeon, joined the 5th Army as a medical commandant. They fought together for France, for their faith in the republic and its justice for all. But it was not the same war as in 1914, and the enemy was not the same *Boche,* though again the Germans had set out on a murderous rampage for world domination. Weeks stretched into months as French troops sat along the Maginot Line of defense on the eastern border, waiting for battle. When it finally came, with a sudden storm of blitzkrieg on May 10, 1940, the power and speed of the German troops stunned the French army. The Germans surged through the Netherlands, Belgium, Luxembourg, and then into eastern France in a matter of days, backed by aerial bombing and heavy artillery. Seven German armored divisions smashed through the Ardennes Forest to take the French town of Sedan. There was no need to destroy the supposedly impenetrable Maginot Line defenses: they simply went around them. At the same time, civilians who lived in the targeted areas raced westward to escape the onslaught, pushing wooden carts, piling into cars, walking with all the possessions they could carry in their arms. It was a humanitarian disaster of extraordinary proportions: an estimated 8 to 10 million refugees were running to nowhere, equipped with nothing, riding a mounting wave of public panic. They had seen newsreels of the bombing of Spanish towns in the recent Civil War; they had heard stories of atrocities dusted off from the last war, babies killed, women raped. They fled.

During those six weeks of false hope that became known as the Battle of France, many doctors worked nonstop at thousands of field hospitals across the country. The plan for care of the wounded had ballooned the nation's 20,000 beds to more than 400,000, with clinics set up in casinos, hotels, schools, and army barracks.[2] Even the American Hospital of Paris (AHP), a private hospital in the suburb of Neuilly-sur-Seine, set up three field hospitals and a volunteer ambulance corps. Long before war was declared, the AHP board of governors had drawn up a plan to evacuate civilian patients to field hospitals to make room for military casualties, in coordination with the French Army Medical Service. Their first patient arrived on September 26, 1939, followed by a steady stream that culminated in the overwhelming chaos of the refugee exodus and the collapse of France. The AHP had earned its reputation as a solid partner in aiding France during WWI, when American volunteers showed up to serve as ambulance drivers, nurses, and doctors long before the United States entered the war. In 1914, the ambulance drivers often were college students, many from elite universities such as Harvard and Yale, and teams of doctors from top American hospitals spent months-long rotations treating French wounded. In 1939, the French military command insisted on putting medical services under its control; by then it had the equipment and personnel for transport. Nonetheless, the American Hospital organized a team of women ambulance drivers to ferry patients between Neuilly and its field hospitals. It was awarded a Croix de Guerre citation for its work, one of thirty-three civilian institutions thus honored. Aid funds and refugee assistance centers also were set up by private associations: as in the last war, the US government stayed officially neutral in the early years of the European fray.

Yet the sudden collapse and flight of refugees drew some medical personnel into the vortex of panic. More than 235 medical staff fled their posts in Paris, including nineteen doctors who led medical departments in hospitals. Some were sanctioned after the war. Such was the disorder at the Archangel Hospital in Orsay, a town thirty kilometers southwest of Paris, that some of its medical staff were later prosecuted on criminal charges. With all its hospital directors and doctors already disappeared into the exodus, a nurse asked a passing army doctor what to do with seven patients who could not be transported. He told her to give them fatal doses of morphine. When the other patients and staff were loaded into taxis to flee the approaching Germans, four nurses injected the patients, although one reduced the dose, inadvertently saving the patient, and another of the patients died of a stroke before the morphine took effect. The nurses were charged with voluntary manslaughter and convicted in a 1942 trial, but their lawyer managed to paint the circumstances of the June panic in such vivid terms that their five-year prison terms were suspended. The army doctor whose orders they had followed was never identified.[3]

Most of the estimated thirty thousand American residents of Paris also fled the capital. By June 1940, the US Embassy counted fewer than one thousand Americans still in the country. At that time, with the United States taking an officially neutral position, Americans were under no specific threat. United States Ambassador William C. Bullitt had been asked by the French government, fleeing south days before the Germans arrived in the capital, to declare Paris an open city, in order to avoid further bombing and artillery damage. A bombing attack on the city on June 3 had left more than 250 persons dead and 650 wounded. Then on June 10, the US State Department ordered Bullitt to follow the French government to safety. He refused.

"The fact that I am here is a strong element in preventing a fatal panic," he telegraphed to President Roosevelt in reply. "Remember Gouverneur Morris and his wooden leg in the Terror, Washburne in the Commune, Herrick [in WWI]. It will mean something always to the French and to the Foreign Service that we do not leave though others do. Following in French: *J'y suis. J'y reste.* End French."[4] The US Embassy chargé d'affaires Robert Murphy, by Bullitt's side in Paris, later noted: "This was an extraordinary time demanding unorthodox methods."[5]

The Germans entered Paris on the morning of June 14, 1940, and the German command staff requisitioned several of the finer hotels for headquarters. Ambassador Bullitt negotiated a guarantee of respect for Americans and their property, posting some seven hundred "American property" notices on business and residential doors around the city. The French hoped it was just a waiting game, that as in the previous war, the Americans would join the side of the Allies and tip the balance their way. But some were not willing to wait. On the eve of the German takeover of Paris, Dr. Thierry de Martel, chief surgeon of the American Hospital, took his own life, saying he could not bear to witness the fall of the city he loved. He had fought the Germans in WWI, and had lost his son in that war. He sent a note to Bullitt, who had been a friend: "When I said I would stay in Paris I spoke the truth, but I would have had to add in front of all those gentlemen 'alive or dead,' which would have sounded pretentious. But from the first day of the war I decided to disappear if the Germans entered Paris. As I am pressed by the time (it is already four in the morning) I will simply say that Martel alive is a cashable check, while Martel dead is a check without provision."[6] He was found in his Paris apartment the following day.

Martel's unflagging care during the Battle of France had drawn the admiration of many American Hospital patients, including British airman Paul Richey, shot down over France in May 1940, who dedicated his war memoir *Fighter Pilot* to Martel. "Now that the wounded were coming in, de Martel and [Neal] Rogers operated day after day, continuously from seven in the morning until four the following one," Richey wrote. "The other doctors

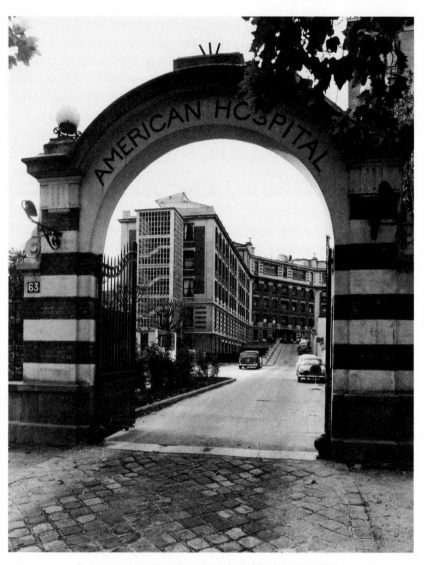

Entrance to the American Hospital of Paris in the 1930s.
American Hospital of Paris archives.

were just as indefatigable, and the nurses never lacked courage, energy or good humour. I thought they were all magnificent, and I am forever indebted to them for their kindness to me."[7]

Marshal Philippe Pétain, an eighty-four-year-old national hero from the First World War and newly named prime minister, announced in a radio broadcast on June 17 that France would surrender to Germany. By then, some sixty thousand French soldiers had died and 1.5 million had been taken prisoner. Pétain's announcement was met with tears by some and with determination by others: French Army Brigadier General Charles de Gaulle, having slipped out of France just before the surrender, announced that he would organize troops to continue the fight. His group became the "Free French" opposition, which would eventually mount an army and fight its way to victory across Africa and then France.

For the surrender, Hitler insisted on the document being signed in the same train car used for the WWI armistice, which he had considered humiliating to Germany, and so top military commanders met on June 22 outside Compiègne. France was divided into zones, with the Atlantic and north coasts and the eastern border forbidden to travel; the northern and western two-thirds under German administration and military command, and the southern third an unoccupied zone. The southeastern borderlands were occupied by the Italian Fascist government allied with the Nazis. In the Unoccupied Zone, French leaders negotiated maintaining an "independent" government in the central spa town of Vichy, whose many hotels made it possible to gather officials from Paris and provincial capitals. On July 10, the National Assembly voted to annul the constitution of the nation's Third Republic and hand all power to Marshal Pétain. Pétain imposed a deeply conservative authoritarian regime on the French, all the while evoking German directions to do so. His pretense was as shallow as his enthusiasm for Nazi measures ran deep.

Ambassador Bullitt wrote in a telegram to Washington on July 1 that he had met with Pétain and his advisers, as well as with military commanders and senators. "The impression which emerges from these conversations is the extraordinary one that the French leaders desire to cut loose from all that France has represented during the past two generations, that their physical and moral defeat has been so absolute that they have accepted completely for France the fate of becoming a province of Nazi Germany," he wrote.[8] Pétain assured Bullitt that the Germans would work with, not against, the French people, that it was in their interest to create an economic "collaboration." Bullitt wrote: "He did not believe that the Germans would break the terms of the armistice and he thought that they would on the contrary do everything to obtain the good will of the people of France and their cooperation in a subordinate role."

On July 11, Bullitt left for the United States, where he resigned as ambassador to France. He did not stick around to see just how wrong Marshal Pétain would be. Many French and foreigners who could get an exit visa out of France did so, sailing from Marseilles. Those without legal options traversed the Pyrénées Mountains into Spain. Lisbon, in neutral Portugal, was a busy point of departure westward during 1940–41.

Jews had particular motive to leave, given the Nazi persecution in Germany and across Eastern Europe, and rising antisemitism in France. In 1940, at the start of the Vichy regime, the Paris area had counted some 150,000 Jewish inhabitants, but within a year the number had dropped to 93,000, a third fewer.[9] Doctors and scientists were among those who swiftly found ways and means to depart. One example is the eminent research Institute of Physico-Chemical Biology, founded by Baron Edmond de Rothschild, later slated for takeover by the Vichy government as a center for eugenics research. Its director noted in a letter of protest that since July 1940, the institute's Jewish doctors and researchers had all left for the United States and Latin America. As early as July 1940, a team of French scientists wrote to ask the Rockefeller Foundation and its New School of Social Research to open positions for French scientists in danger of persecution, traveling to New York in August when their plea went unanswered. The New School eventually requested entry to the United States for three hundred European intellectuals. The Vichy government approved exit visas for some Jewish scientists until April 1941, when a new law forbade men between seventeen and forty years old from leaving France.[10]

Others, sifting through the debris of the surrender, made arrangements to leave immediately. Future Nobel laureate François Jacob, still in medical school, left the country and joined the Free French in London in June 1940. Two months later, he was a medical auxiliary officer in the Free French Army in Dakar, Senegal. Alexandre Krementchousky, a Russian-born, French-trained doctor, also was one of the early adherents to the Free French. Krementchousky was Russian Orthodox, not Jewish, but he didn't wait around. Another Paris practitioner, Dr. André Lichtwitz, scrawled "Gone to fight" across his office door and escaped through Spain to join the Free French in London. The three were among thirty-six doctors named *Compagnons de la Libération,* of a total 1,038 persons distinguished for their early actions against the occupier.

As soon as they took over, German authorities requisitioned four of the region's best-equipped hospitals for German troops only, barring French patients. Beaujon Hospital was newly constructed in 1935 in the Paris suburb of Clichy, and Lariboisière Hospital, which had opened in the Tenth Arrondissement of Paris in 1854 after a cholera epidemic, counted more than one thousand beds by the early twentieth century. The third hospital the Germans took was La Pitié, an early seventeenth-century children's hospice for beggars and orphans; it had merged with the Salpêtrière hospice for women in 1657, becoming one of the largest institutions of its kind in Europe. The Pitié-Salpêtrière complex had become a teaching hospital in the early twentieth century, with a specialty in neurology and psychiatry. And the Hôpital Foch, in the western suburb of Suresnes, was built in the 1930s with the help of donations from a Franco-American foundation and two American women of considerable fortune, Consuelo Vanderbilt and Winnaretta Singer. There were still in the Paris area 120 other hospitals, clinics, hospices, and medical centers operating in the centralized Public Assistance (AP) network, which treated some 150,000 patients either in facilities or at home and employed some 35,000 health professionals.[11]

Jews and foreigners among the AP medical staff were soon targeted by new rules drawn up by the Vichy government. Issued in July 1940, the measures expelled from public administration positions—including doctors in the public health service—anyone whose father was not French, regardless of previous naturalization. An exception would be made for those who had fought for France in 1914–18 or in 1939–40. A month later, the ban was extended to private professional practice, whether in medicine, law, architecture, or notarial services. Also excluded were any Freemasons of the secretive fraternal order. In the Paris region, the Préfecture of Police produced a list of 915 doctors out of an estimated total of six thousand, or 15 percent of practitioners, who fell into this new non-French category. Of them, 567 requested an exemption to avoid being forced out. While their cases were under review, they could continue to work.[12]

Campaigning against so-called foreigners was a classic method of stirring up the resentment and hatred of nativist reaction. Added to the global economic crash, a downturn that reached France in 1931, lawmakers had found wide support for measures limiting the number of foreign medical students and doctors, or assigning long waiting periods before their practice was approved. These measures, contained in the Armbruster Law of 1933 and the Cousin-Nast Law of 1935, came into application just as the Nazis and their allies in Eastern Europe blocked Jews from schools, professions, public venues, and more, sending increasing numbers of refugees westward.[13] In the mid- to late 1930s, the majority of the foreigners in the Paris Medical School were Romanian, Polish, and Russian immigrants, many of them Jews. Thus Vichy's move to exclude foreigners was little more than an early foundation for its subsequent anti-Jewish laws. Their effect on medical practice in France was immediate and devastating, as discussed in chapter 2.

It is difficult to separate public medical practice from public health, and Occupation restrictions on food and medicine undermined both. The French found all safety nets—social, economic, and political—had been destroyed and the most basic need of all—food—was threatened. Food rationing had been imposed in March 1940, three months before the surrender, as the war footing reduced production. By August, patients had to bring their own ration cards to hospital in order to be fed, and the rest of the population was put on a strict diet. The Vichy government created six categories of consumers: E (children 0–3 years old); J1 and J2 (children 3–12); J3 (adolescents 13–21); A (adults), and V (70 or more years old). Base rations amounted to between 1,200 and 1,800 calories a day, with a little extra for heavy laborers and pregnant women. This already minimal level was cut again in 1943 to 1,100 calories a day. That represents about half of today's medical recommendation: 2,000 calories a day for a woman and 2,500 for a man. Finding food, from black-market or other sources, became an obsession. The widespread lack of nutrition sent disease levels soaring, stunted children's growth, and brought death to those in fragile health. Historians have estimated that 95,000 persons in hospices and prisons died of hunger during the Occupation, bringing the death rate to 17 percent of the population (compared with .9 percent today).[14]

In a 1945 essay trying to explain what the Occupation had been like, Jean-Paul Sartre, the writer and philosopher who had remained in Paris through the war, described hunger and food as the last rock to stand on in the floodwaters of despair. "Our requirements diminished along with our memory, and, as people become accustomed to everything, we suffered the shame of getting used to our misery, to the Swedish turnips that were served us, to the minimal liberties still left us, and to the barrenness within us. Each day our ways became simpler, and we finally reached a point where we spoke only of food, less out of hunger or fear of the morrow, perhaps, than because the pursuit of food was the only activity of which we were still capable."[15]

Conditions of want, misery, and oppression did not bring out the best in everyone. Many people struggled for their daily (soon ersatz) bread, and while they resented the German Occupation, they kept their focus on survival. After the war, historians identified four general groups of French reaction to the Occupation. They qualified about 100,000 French as active collaborators who worked with the Nazis out of ideological conviction. They were the smallest group. In the middle, the largest two groups were those who accommodated the new masters and perhaps even thrived, and then those who adapted, who changed the way they lived but avoided exchange with the Germans. The last group, a minority of perhaps 300,000, was composed of those who devoted themselves to active resistance, who gave up their comfort and security to take action against the occupier.[16] Who were the doctors among them?

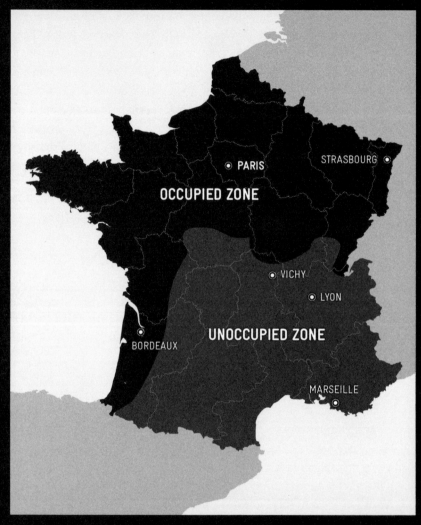

Map of France, demarcation between Occupied and Unoccupied Zones, 1941.
Anastasia Komnou.

2

THE RACIALIZATION
OF HATRED

For all the differences between the First World War and the Second, the strongest element of change was the racialization of hatred. The Nazi Germans had drawn a profile of superiority based on a prescribed "Aryan" model: white, heterosexual, conservative, Christian— though not religious. Anyone whose identity fell outside the mold was a potential victim of repression, imprisonment, or death. In order to rank social groups on a vertical scale, all people had to be categorized by race and identified by ancestry. The mania to which they subscribed is evident in a scheme drawn up by a Nazi collaborator: the "French race" was divided geographically into four "sub-races," all declared "Aryan." Africans, Slavs, and Roma were persecuted based on race and identity, while homosexuals, Jehovah's Witnesses, and common criminals were punished as "asocial" types. But above and beyond all the others, the Nazis' primary targets of racial hatred were Jews. The persecution of Jews carried out in Germany quickly made its way to France with the Occupation, receiving a warm welcome from some of the French. Many of those who scurried to work for the Vichy government did so in order to express their antisemitism from a position of power.

Antisemitic rumbling had been intensifying through the 1930s across Eastern Europe, then Germany and France. In Germany, Jewish doctors were excluded from practicing medicine in 1933, when Adolf Hitler took office as chancellor, and allied governments in Poland, Romania, and Hungary followed suit. This led to a wave of emigration westward, with France often the first stop. Some 175,000 to 200,000 Jewish immigrants had moved to France by 1939, bringing the Jewish population to an estimated 330,000 in a population of 41 million, not more than 1 percent.[1] Far larger immigrant groups in France at that time were Italians, Poles, and Spaniards, who numbered around 2 million. And France needed immigrant workers to fill the shoes of the generation—1.4 million men—lost in the Great War. In broadly general terms, Italians and Spaniards mostly stayed in the south, working in agriculture, while Poles went to the north, to the coal mines. An estimated two-thirds of Jewish immigrants settled in Paris, working in commerce or liberal professions.[2] Then, as now, fearmongers dismissed positive aspects of immigration in favor of stirring up hatred and resentment.

Anti-immigration organizations and press announced in 1936 that Jews had comprised 15 percent of doctors licensed to practice in French public hospitals in 1929, and that by 1936 they represented 35 percent of the total. These figures were hugely exaggerated: the government finally released the actual figures in 1938, showing that foreigners numbered 319 of 5,636 doctors—just 5 percent—in Paris-region hospitals.[3] While Jews were among the ranks of foreign doctors, they were not the entire bloc, a fact also elided by the antisemitic campaigners. But the racist voices were loud, their publications many, and competition for the limited number of hospital practitioners was steep. Even prior to the 1930s, associations of medical students and medical unions demanded a ceiling quota for foreigners, and about half the Jews in France fell into that category. In 1933, with public opinion sharpening against immigration, the French Assembly passed the Armbruster Law, requiring both a French medical diploma and French citizenship (previously one or the other had sufficed) in order to practice. In 1935, the Cousin-Nast Law added a five-year waiting period for foreign-born doctors who qualified for public hospital practice.

Thus before the Germans occupied France, before the Vichy government began churning out its imitation-Nazi policies, the French government had instituted measures against foreigners in medicine. The laws were not specifically against Jews; several non-Jewish American doctors who wanted to practice in France were obliged to take the exams as well, starting with the high-school *baccalauréat.*

Then, with the ink barely dry on the surrender, a short-lived law against public or press attacks arousing hatred against people based on their race or religion was repealed.[4] Jews were hit with unrelenting and vicious attacks in the French press, which under the Vichy government became either archconservative or clandestine. There were a dozen daily newspapers and a half-dozen weeklies published in France whose columns praised Pétain, slammed the British, and excoriated Jews. From July 1940, the weekly *Au Pilori* (To the Pillory), subsidized by the German propaganda office, spewed hatred in headlines that were aimed specifically at Jews and Freemasons. Its subtitle was "Weekly Combat Against Judeo-Masonry" (*"Hebdomadaire de Combat Contre la Judeo-Maçonnerie"*). It didn't take long to target Jewish doctors. On August 10, 1940, the first article to attack doctors appeared under the headline "Let's Purify France (*Epurons la France*)." It listed fifteen hospitals and three medical institutes that employed more than thirty doctors it identified as Jewish. The list continued in the following issue, with a note explaining that if anyone brought proof of Aryan ascendancy they could be removed from the list. "We repeat that we reject any argument on religious grounds and only racial identification is of interest," the editors wrote.[5] In other words, the practice of one religion or the other was not relevant; what mattered to the new powers was heredity.

Among the doctors on *Au Pilori*'s list was the pediatrician Robert Debré, a slight, elegant WWI veteran who practiced in Paris hospitals. Debré was six years old when he moved to Neuilly-sur-Seine, a quiet riverside town on the western edge of Paris, after his father was named assistant rabbi to the Paris synagogue in 1888. Simon Debré, one of a long line of Alsatian rabbis, had taken French nationality in 1872 while in high school. The Germans had annexed Alsace in the 1870 Franco-Prussian war, at which point many Alsatians moved across the border to French territory. Simon Debré had earned a rabbinical degree and had officiated in the French town of Sedan, while in the evenings teaching German to French officers stationed there. During the First World War, he had served as chaplain to the French Army while his three sons were on active duty, and after the war he was named chief rabbi of Neuilly and chevalier in the prestigious Legion of Honor. Robert had grown up in a religious home, flanked by two brothers, a sister, and his childhood neighbor and friend, the future Swedish consul Raoul Nordling. He and Nordling were schoolmates at the prominent Lycée Janson-de-Sailly, where Simon Debré served as chaplain, along with two Catholic priests and a Protestant pastor. School curriculum was entirely secular, with religious study offered after class.

Robert Debré graduated from medical school in 1906, married in 1908, had three children and began a career in the medical care of children, a fairly recent specialty. He served as a military doctor in the Great War, so when the second round broke out in 1939, he added a few stripes to his old uniform and went to the Health Ministry to help organize the military medical services. In May 1940, he joined troops moving eastward, witnessing the disintegration of the Ninth French Army at the Meuse River. He returned to Paris and followed the government to Bordeaux, and then to Vichy. After the surrender, he was told it would be dangerous for him, as a Jew, to return to Paris. It was meant as a friendly warning, to keep him safe. But Robert Debré was not one to turn away from a challenge or back down from a threat. He resolved to return to Paris and to represent in his own life and work a contrary example to the malicious anti-Jewish propaganda being sown.

First, he had to help his eldest son, Michel, age twenty-seven, being held in a prisoner-of-war camp at Autun by the Germans. He went to the camp and found his son in a barbed-wire cage, beaten and isolated for having tried to escape. Debré and friends drew up a plan to get him out, and by September 4, Michel was free and hiding in the family's country house in the Loire Valley. Michel Debré eventually joined the Resistance and would become the first prime minister of the Fifth Republic under President Charles de Gaulle. Robert's daughter, Claude, twenty-six, was in medical school in Paris, and his son Olivier, nineteen, was an architecture student at the Ecole de Beaux Arts. Robert Debré went home to his apartment at 5 rue de l'Université in the Seventh Arrondissement. "Paris! Paris at last, Paris forever, but Paris in shame," he wrote in a private journal he kept throughout the war.[6] It was September, classes were starting again at the University of Paris Medical School, where he was chairman of bacteriology; the elite Academy of Medicine had begun meeting again, and he was developing a pediatrics service at the Herold Hospital in northeast Paris. He was busy, but found the atmosphere in Paris "morally intolerable." German soldiers were everywhere, the red-and-black swastika flew from public buildings, signs were in German. It started out ugly, and would only get worse.

On October 3, France's Vichy government issued its first anti-Jewish laws (*le Statut des Juifs*), first defining who would be considered as Jewish: anyone with three Jewish grandparents or two Jewish grandparents and a Jewish spouse. It then banned Jews from positions of government or public administration, military command, the press, film and theater, or teaching, allowing for an exemption if they had served in or been decorated for military service during 1914–18 or 1939–40. Doctors and medical professionals were not named specifically in this first strike, but on October 30, the direc-

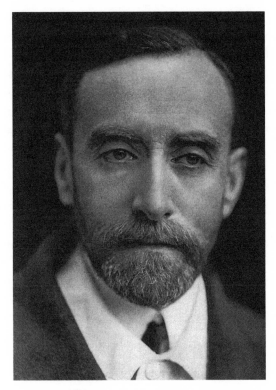

Dr. Robert Debré in the early 1930s.
BIU Santé médecine—Université Paris Cité.

tors of the Public Assistance hospital network sent a memo to its institutions. Anyone meeting the definition given in the new law must resign immediately from their position.

Debré did not expect the interdiction to apply to him. He did not consider himself a religious man and had left Judaism behind. As a teenager, he announced to his father that he had weighed science against religion and decided on the side of science. He would not go to temple any more. It was deeply painful to his father, a breach they perhaps did not ever repair, but Robert was adamant. He carried his conviction through to a preparatory science school and then to medical school. Two years later, he married one of the few women in his medical school class. Jeanne Debat-Ponson was the brilliant daughter of an artist, from a Catholic family, and like Debré, more inclined to science than to religion. Both their families opposed the marriage, and both watched it flourish in the years to come.[7]

He continued treating patients in hospitals and at homes, as well as teaching a few hours a day, as doctors did in French hospitals at the time. But in December, Debré was asked to resign from his teaching position at the Medical School. He noted in his journal: "Appalled by this Jewish problem, nauseated to keep getting stuck in it. Feels like an obsessive nightmare, impossible to escape." When the fact of his Jewish heritage became the primary obstacle to his work, Debré was doubly frustrated. Then, also in December, when his name was removed from the list of doctors certified to practice in French public hospitals, he could make no more rounds of patients. As he left, the medical staff of Necker-Enfants Malades Hospital crowded into the amphitheater to say goodbye. He gave a short speech: "I will return. You, my friends, continue to work!"[8] People wrote protests on his behalf, even his friend the renowned poet Paul Valéry wrote to Marshal Pétain, lauding Debré's accomplishments in medicine as well as his service in the First World War. Pétain's response to this individual case paralleled his attitude toward the nation. He wrote to Valéry on December 20, 1940: "I have imposed upon myself the discipline of not personally intervening for anyone, wishing to leave to the commissions assigned to study these cases the entire liberty of their judgment." The letter continued: "Despite all desire to be agreeable, I can do nothing, though the great services rendered by Professor Debré should be recognized, as I am aware he is one of the luminaries of French science."[9] There was a rumor, Valéry was told unofficially, that Debré had said the Marshal should be shot. True, or false? Debré neither confirmed nor denied.

At Parisian society dinner parties, listening to loud advice for acquiescence to the Occupation, Debré heard self-interest at work. "Except for [Henri] Mondor and I, they curse the English, they talk of collaboration, of arrangements with Germany, they are ready for any concessions, they have finished their grieving for national integrity, they abandon Alsace and Lorraine, they consider other [territorial] amputations and they say: 'Let's negotiate quickly, before the English do.' I shudder at these words, which seem to me to betray faith in the nation and represent the most calculating falseness ever," he wrote.[10]

In June 1941, the General Commission on Jewish Questions, a Vichy agency created a few months before to direct its antisemitic policies, began issuing revised legislation that in August imposed a ceiling quota on native-born Jews from private-sector professions such as medicine, law, architecture, and pharmacies. They had been pushed out of public positions in government or teaching, removed from commerce, and now were forced out of liberal professions as well. The newly created Medical Order (*Ordre des Médecins*) was told to cap the number of Jewish doctors at 2 percent of the total. Working from a Seine Department (Paris region) 1939 census that counted some 900 Jewish doctors among a total of 5,410, the Order was told to select 110 Jewish doctors who could continue to work, while nearly 800 had two months to close up shop or to apply for an exemption.[11] Exemptions could be given for those who were decorated veterans of WWI, or whose skills could not be found elsewhere. As noted previously, 567 doctors already had applied for an exemption to the antiforeigner measures.

The Medical Order had been formed to establish professional standards in areas such as setting fees, naming medical conditions, and prescribing treatment—and now its first task would be to block Jewish doctors from practicing, even privately. Dr. René Leriche, an eminent vascular surgeon, was named president of the Medical Order's Superior Council by the Vichy government in October 1940. Alsatian by birth, Leriche wrote in a 1956 memoir that he was told by the Vichy minister who appointed him he could consider his position as a vindication of the Germans' takeover of his region. Leriche wrote he had tried to avoid an appointment with Vichy, but feared he would be saddled with a worse position if he refused. These postwar excuses were not the whole truth. In fact, he had written letters lobbying for the post in August 1940 to Dr. Bernard Ménétrel, personal physician and secretary to Marshal Pétain. He was determined to lead a reorganization and modernization of the medical profession in France. "I have become convinced of the necessity of a complete reform, in spirit and in fact," he wrote on August 25. "Those who undertake these questions must share a conviction: that of the increasingly declining influence of French medicine in the world. Contrary to what the French too easily believe, our role in the development of ideas has come to a halt."[12] Doctors had been trying to form a professional association since the mid-nineteenth century, and Leriche was interested in developing medical protocols for patient care along with standardizing doctors' compensation and retirement benefits. He did not mention Jewish doctors in his correspondence, but wrote an effusive note thanking Marshal Pétain for the opportunity to lead the Medical Order. For the first few months, the Medical Order worked on developing professional standards. It also was assigned to certify and publish lists of Order-approved doctors practicing in each region and department. The conservative *Concours Médical* newspaper, which counted some eleven thousand readers, hammered the point about non-French doctors taking advantage of the nation's generosity, and demanded that exclusions be effected rapidly. The magazine printed a copy of the questionnaire doctors had to complete in order to be approved. The first few questions focused on birthplace, nationality and parents' nationalities, rather than medical education.[13]

Through the spring of 1941, lists of names of "foreign" doctors who were forbidden to practice were published in the Medical Order's Bulletin, and also by regional medical councils. The large majority were of Romanian descent, most of them Jewish. For the Medical Order, Leriche wrote that he would slow down the exclusions as much as possible, conducting lengthy investigations into each individual and applying for exemptions wherever there was potential for success. His method worked to the extent that the Medical Order was loudly criticized in the Vichy press, called a "judeo-masonic citadel" that catered to Jewish and immigrant interests. *Au Pilori* opined that if Jewish doctors could not be removed, the government's Commissioner for Jewish Questions should resign. The Medical Order's Council explained its actions in a report in the *Bulletin de l'Ordre des Médecins,* saying it was obliged to obey the law, but had tried to get as many exemptions from removal as possible, "based on the eminent character of their services and their professional merit."[14]

On the other side, doctors were suspicious that the Medical Order was little more than a tool for the Vichy government to control the medical profession. In the clandestine newsletter *Le Médecin français* (The French Doctor), begun by two practitioners in March 1941, a writer complained in April 1942 that Dr. Leriche's excuses for the Medical Order being unable to counter antisemitic measures were evidence of Vichy's bad faith. "It demonstrates that the Order Council is powerless to fulfill any role other than as factotum of the Vichy government, and that Vichy, a Hitlerian government, doesn't give a damn about the needs of French doctors. Professor Leriche confesses implicitly that we are correct."[15]

Despite Pétain's sworn disinterest, the Vichy government did come through on January 5, 1941, with an exemption from the anti-Jewish statutes for Robert Debré, along with nine other prominent scholars and scientists. "Considering that Doctor Robert Debré is, in the subject of pediatrics, a master whose reputation is universal; that his work on infantile maladies, notably cerebrospinal meningitis, measles, diphtheria and tuberculosis, is at the origin of notable progress in the knowledge and treatment of these diseases [. . .], he is exempted from the interdictions brought by the law of October 3, 1940."[16] Nowhere does the declaration mention the word "Jew," and what seemed a typographical error—the decree will be *oublié* (forgotten) instead of *publié* (published)—turned into a six-month wait for the decree to appear in the *Journal Officiel,* an act required for it to go into effect. The Vichy education minister, Jérôme Carcopino, had pushed for the exemptions, and the German military command had pushed back, expressing formal opposition. Nonetheless, in July 1941, the exemptions were published in the *Journal Officiel.* Carcopino wrote to tell Debré he would continue to receive his professor's salary but asked that he not try to teach at the Paris Medical School. By then, Debré was the only one of the ten exempted men remaining in Paris. "[He] would not dream of moving his patients to the provinces," Carcopino wrote, somewhat archly, in his memoir.[17]

While Paris was far from the safest roost, the fate of the other nine scholars traces no pattern of distance providing shelter. Three scholars moved south and taught at universities in the Unoccupied Zone until 1943 or 1944, when they had to go into hiding to avoid arrest. Two other exemptees joined the Resistance and were eventually arrested and executed by German troops. One scholar was deported to Auschwitz and survived, while another was sent to Drancy in August 1944, just weeks before it was liberated, and survived. Two others escaped to the United States.[18]

In the meantime, Debré and Dr. Gaston Nora, also under exclusion as a Jew, went to see Xavier Vallat, a man known for his hardline views and blaring antisemitism, who had been named head of the General Commission on Jewish Questions. Vallat was a veteran of the Great War, wounded by artillery in 1914 and again in 1915, then lost an eye to infection in 1916, and despite each injury, had returned voluntarily to fighting at the front. Then, in combat in 1918, Vallat's leg was blown up by a grenade. As he lay on the ground under intense artillery fire, a young medic from his infantry company dashed out to drag him to safety. It was Gaston Nora, and after the war, the two men continued their combat-born camaraderie, until Vallat was elected to the National Assembly. As a right-wing congressman in the 1930s, Vallat's antisemitic rants drove a wedge in their relations. That afternoon in his office in Saint-Germain-des-Prés, Vallat listened to Nora and Debré appeal to his sense of patriotism, but he was unmoved. After they left, Nora and Debré compared impressions. "Neither heart nor intelligence," diagnosed Debré.[19]

Debré and Nora were among twenty or so prominent Jewish veterans of WWI who signed a letter to Marshal Pétain protesting against the exclusionary measures. They included an Army general, an industrialist, lawyers, and several doctors. "We form neither a race nor a people, but an integral part of the Nation, from which nothing will be able to separate us," they wrote. The letter made a strong appeal to a sense of patriotism, which Pétain had been known to possess in the past. "The Jews of France, those who have had the honor to serve under your orders, in the armies, those whose sons and brothers have fallen for the well-being of all, those whose parents and ancestors spilled their blood side by side with your parents and your ancestors for the defense of the ground of France—yours and theirs—will they now see themselves hit with the hardest blow of all, and excluded, pell-mell, from the national sovereignty?"[20]

Dr. André Cain, also a decorated WWI veteran and French citizen, had managed to stay on as chief of gastroenterology at Saint Antoine Hospital in Paris, until the Gestapo called him in for a long and chilling interrogation in September 1941. The rabid press had referred to his hospital as "the synagogue Saint-Antoine" because of the number of Jews practicing there. Cain had gone on staff at Saint Antoine shortly after the Great War, in which he was awarded a Croix de Guerre citation for bravery, and served again in 1939–40 as a commandant in the army's medical corps. His director had issued a commendation for his courage in 1940: "Your attitude is a lesson to those who, without orders or despite orders received, fled before the enemy, forgetting their professional duty."[21]

Cain had known when to stand firm and hold his ground. But now, with the Gestapo on his back, it was time to go. He and his wife packed up and fled to the south immediately, followed by their daughter and son-in-law, along with their two children. The Cains's son Pierre had been in medical school in Marseille until he was expelled as a Jew, so they went there first, and then eventually the family moved to Lyon. While the southern zone was less overtly policed in the early Occupation, spies and traitors abounded. With the German takeover of the zone in November 1942, many of those who had sought refuge there took on false identities or tried to emmigrate to surer ground. Cain was undoubtedly aware that any safe harbor there would be temporary. "He crossed the line of demarcation, abandoning everything: his position, hospital service, work underway, and all the familiar objects upon which his gaze would rest, which were completely and entirely pillaged by the Germans," a friend and fellow doctor wrote later.[22] Cain could not find work as a doctor in the south. While the 2 percent ceiling was less of a problem in the provinces than in the Paris area, the designated Jewish slots had been filled.

Yet the exclusions and interdictions were not enough for some. Captain Paul Sézille, secretary general of the Institute for the Study of Jewish Questions, a private, German-sponsored agency created in March 1941 to promote antisemitism, wrote to the health minister in January 1942. Too many Jewish doctors were being given two- to four-month-long postponements of their exclusion, allowing them to continue practicing, he wrote. Sézille wanted to draw the minister's attention to "the dangers that these Jewish doctors represent, these foreigners, who, by their propaganda—because you will not doubt, Mr. Minister, that these Jewish doctors are the enemies of the collaboration and even the government of the Marshal—do great damage to our French families."[23]

Sézille did not know, at that time, the extent to which a handful of Jewish doctors were in fact actively working against the Vichy regime, doing every bit of damage they could to its malignant agenda, and saving countless lives in the process. Sézille, later described as having a violent, alcoholic, antagonistic character, was the darling of the German propagandists for a while, but even they grew tired of his blustery tirades.

3

DANGER TAKES SHAPE

Many of the doctors who decided to stay in Paris did so not because they agreed with the Vichy government or supported the German Occupation, but because their professional, social, and family lives were so deeply embedded in the capital that they could not imagine leaving. In the early part of the Occupation, they continued their usual routines, while keeping an eye on the horizon. For some, the intensifying persecution of Jews, as well as tightening controls over medical privileges and worsening health conditions, motivated them to organize for resistance.

Louis Pasteur Vallery-Radot was the only son of the renowned scientist Louis Pasteur's daughter, Marie-Louise, and René Vallery-Radot, an editor and writer. He adored his grandfather, who had discovered that high temperatures killed bacteria, a life-saving process named pasteurization after him, one among his many important breakthroughs to modernity in medicine. Photographs of young Louis with his grandfather show the same determined chin and steely gaze of confidence. He was nine years old when his grandfather died in 1895, but he carried on his passion for science, focused on medicine. Pasteur Vallery-Radot completed his hospital residency for medical school in 1913, just in time to serve as an army medic in the Great War, and was certified for hospital practice in 1920. When the second war broke out, Pasteur Vallery-Radot—by then fifty-three years old and known widely as PVR—joined the government as a medical adviser and was sent on mission to Indochina. Back in France in June 1940, he huddled in Bordeaux with the rest of the refugee government. When he heard Pétain's June 17 surrender broadcast on the radio, he broke down in tears. The next day, he listened to the BBC as an inspired French Army general, Charles

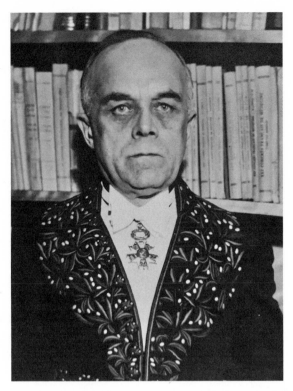

Dr. Louis Pasteur Vallery-Radot, at the Académie Française in 1949.
Bibliothèque Nationale de France.

de Gaulle, urged France to fight on. "Ah! A breath of hope!" he wrote in his memoir.[1]

PVR and his wife, Jacqueline, returned to Paris, a grueling trip that took forty-eight hours and offered no food along the way. Before the war, PVR had given his grandfather's papers to the Institut Pasteur and his possessions to the Musée Pasteur, and in 1940 was named president of the Institut's governing council. He had been elected by his peers to the National Academy of Medicine and named to the board of directors of the Legion of Honor. He was head of a medical department at Bichat Hospital, professor of pathology at the Paris Medical School, and published widely on medical research, as well as writing two biographies of his grandfather. It would have been difficult to have more social and professional status in France in the 1940s than did PVR. He and Jacqueline knew everyone and were invited to dinner everywhere. It was not surprising that the Vichy government tried to get him on board, asking him to serve as head of the French Red Cross. He lasted three months, at which point he could not stomach having to deal with the hardline Vichy bureaucrats any more. He knew Marshal Pétain personally, and when he ran into him, did not hesitate to push him on one point or another concerning the regime. To no avail.

Of the first winter, 1940–41, he wrote: "We spent a sad winter, eating rutabagas and chewing on our shame."[2] Postwar, PVR published *Mémoires d'un non-conformist,* opening fire with a warning: "I am a non-conformist, but I grew up in the most conformist atmosphere there was; my life has been a mix of conformism and emancipated liberty," he wrote. "I loathe people who take themselves seriously. I really don't give a damn."[3] He was not what people expected, and he delighted in being unpredictable. Submitting to the occupying forces, or sitting by while Vichy desecrated the medical community, did not coincide with PVR's character in the least. So when he learned that some of the staff of the Musée de l'Homme (Museum of Mankind) were secretly organizing against the Occupation, PVR leapt at the opportunity. His medical intern and research assistant, Dr. Paul Milliez, was the nephew of Paul Rivet, the museum director and one of the Resistance network founders. Rivet's response to the June 1940 surrender had been to post a copy of Rudyard Kipling's poem *If* above the door to the museum: "If you can keep your head when all about you are losing theirs and blaming it on you . . ." *Au Pilori* complained in a September 1940 article that Rivet had encouraged his staff to raise their fists and boo Hitler during his single visit to Paris on June 23, when he stopped next to the museum at the Place de Trocadero. "We have witnesses," the article said. "He should be fired."[4] Postwar, his profile was put on a medal.

At first, the group watched German activities and movements and reported them to Yvonne Pagniez, one of the organizers, a nurse who had trained in intelligence work in WWI, and who had found a contact to send information on to London. Paul Milliez wrote in his memoirs that it was dangerous and frustrating, as they risked their lives to find things out, and then never heard back whether it was helpful or not. Their only reward, he wrote, was if a factory they had identified as being useful to the Germans then was bombed. Milliez worked closely with PVR, much of his time spent trying to keep his eccentric boss, who tended to tell anyone he met that the Germans would soon be gone, out of trouble. He suggested lowering PVR's profile—he was too well-known in Paris—by disguising him as a Basque peasant, in beret, mustache, and simple clothes. Milliez, who was twenty-eight, noted that he himself wore many disguises during this period. But PVR always showed up in his Lanvin suits. Occupation or no, his style was couture. PVR's wife once remarked as they embarked on their bicycles for another mission that they reminded her of nothing so much as Sancho Panza and Don Quixote.

PVR and Robert Debré were close friends. PVR wrote that they were "inseparable"; they had been young interns under the esteemed professor Fernand Widal, they had fought in the Great War, and then they had traveled side-by-side on an ambitious and socially prominent track to become eminent physicians. Now they found themselves sharing a position of rebellion against authority, against their own government. Individually and together, they weighed whether they could live on the occupier's terms and decided firmly that they could not, regardless of the risk. As a Jew, Debré was in a much more vulnerable position. But he also had seen, as an adolescent, an example of what could be done in the face of antisemitism. He had gotten into the courtroom to watch the scandalous trial of author Emile Zola. In February 1898, Zola was sued by the French Army commander for having explained to the public, in a newspaper article headlined *"J'Accuse,"* the conspiracy mounted by army leaders against Captain Alfred Dreyfus. Dreyfus, an Alsatian Jew like the Debrés, was accused of having sold state secrets to Germany. Debré, even at sixteen years old, knew that that was a ridiculous charge. No Alsatian Jew would betray France for Germany! The "Dreyfus Affair," as it became known, was bitterly controversial at the time, with friends and families taking opposite sides of the case, and antisemitism emerging into public discourse in its ugly way. It was the first time Debré had encountered it.

"It was only during the Dreyfus Affair that we began to hear, during demonstrations and in student roughhousing, the hostile shouts," he wrote.[5] It is a measure of the social integration of the time that Debré, the rabbi's son, was best friends with the son of the vice president of the powerful Council of State, and it was with him and his mother that Debré got into the courtroom for Zola's trial. He remarked on the high-strung tension and utter hostility of the crowd to Zola that day, and said that he and his friends admired the writer endlessly for his courage. Now it was Debré's turn to take a stand in a malevolent tide.

He was not alone. Debré had lost his beloved wife Jeanne in 1929, when she fell ill with a fever and died. He was devastated by her death, and it was not until 1937, with Elisabeth de La Bourdonnaye, that he began a new relationship. He called her Dexia, Greek for right, which she took for her Resistance *nom de guerre*. A forty-two-year-old countess and mother of six, she left her husband for Debré, who had been her children's doctor, and went to work for him as a secretary at Necker Hospital. Her marriage to Alphonse de La Bourdonnaye, an older, staidly conservative landowner, had been arranged when she was nineteen. Her father was General Louis de La Panouse and her mother Sabine de Wendel, of a Lorraine industrialist family, neither of them Jewish, both of them prominent and wealthy. Robert wrote about her constantly in his journal of the time, lunches together, travels, witty comments she made, how wonderful she looked. He was deeply in love.

Both of them were politically committed to opposing the Vichy government and the Nazi Occupation. Yet moving from desire to action was delicate; first approaches to a Resistance group had to be indirect. One conversation bore the result they hoped for. Debré dropped the idea that he would like to be able to "do something" to help France, and separately, Elisabeth offered her apartment on rue de Varenne, should anyone need a place to stay.[6] They were talking to Boris Vildé, ethnologist at the Musée de l'Homme, who had founded with Paul Rivet and some coworkers the "National Committee of Public Health," known to history as the Musée de l'Homme group. Vildé said he needed places to hide young men seeking to flee Vichy and join the Free French in London. Chanterac, the La Bourdonnaye castle in the southwestern woods of the Dordogne, provided a secluded spot to await passage over the Pyrénées Mountains to Spain. Elisabeth's eldest son, Geoffroy, and a group of English, Polish, and French soldiers, along with two women nurses, escaped through that route in November 1940. Vildé suggested to Debré that he could write short tracts countering Vichy propaganda, analyzing events from a different point of view. Such anonymous, typewritten papers could be left casually in public places. It helped, Vildé said, for people to hear from sources other than the government and its media mouthpieces. Debré was happy to comply. Elisabeth did the typing.

In December 1940, the group began publishing the four-to-six page news sheet they called "Résistance." The name came from the museum's librarian, Yvonne Oddon, who recalled the fate of some Protestant women following the 1585 Revocation of the Edict of Nantes. After they were imprisoned for continuing to practice their faith, one of them famously scratched "Résist" on the stone walls of her cell. Oddon wrote in a later memoir: "I couldn't help but remember the word engraved long ago on the walls of the Tower of Constance by a group of Huguenot 'resistants' and it seemed to me to exactly translate our state of mind. Because at the beginning, the underlying reason for all our acts was less a feeling of rebellion that an affirmation of faith."[7]

Her choice of words echoed those by General Charles de Gaulle, in his speech over the BBC on June 18, 1940: "Whatever happens, the flame of French resistance must not be extinguished and will not be extinguished."[8]

The daughter of an army officer who died of wounds from WWI, Oddon had studied at the American Library School in Paris and then worked at the US Library of Congress in the 1930s. When Rivet began his project of transforming the old Ethnography Museum into the Museum of Mankind, Oddon took over the library and constructed a documentation and research center. During the German Occupation, she used her contacts at the US Embassy to get information to print in the news sheet, whose masthead carried a quote from Napoleon Bonaparte: "To live in defeat is to die every day."[9]

The Musée de l'Homme network also began helping to hide British and French aviators who had been shot down over Occupied territory. Several escape-and-evasion lines had sprung up from the need to hide the airmen in France and get them safely across the Spanish border or the English Channel. Paul Milliez worked with Robert Aylé, one of the founders of the legendary Comet escape-and-evasion line, in Paris in the early days. In one episode, Milliez had obtained a list of Paris police officers and their political leanings—who could be called on for help?—and met Aylé, both on bicycles, when suddenly they were boxed in on the Pont de la Concorde, German soldiers blocking either end. Milliez thought they were done for, but Aylé, cool as could be, approached and asked a soldier to let them through. Off they went, list safely in hand.[10]

With its success, the Musée de l'Homme network grew until it counted more than one hundred members. And with growth came danger. Not from the Germans, they were easily detected and avoided. French infiltrators, secret agents of the Gestapo who pretended to be on the side of the Resistance, worked to gain the confidence of network members, and then handed them over to imprisonment or death. Two of the most sordid traitors of the war, Albert Gaveau and Jacques Desoubrie, did just that to the Musée de l'Homme network in early 1941. They were aided by two Russian neighbors of Yvonne Oddon, also employees of the museum, who had persuaded her they wanted to help the Resistance. In fact, they were working undercover

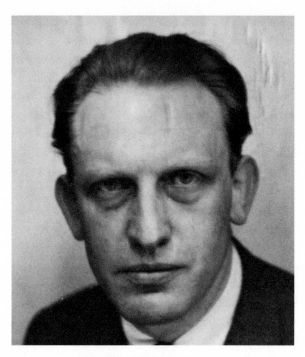

Dr. Paul Milliez in the 1940s.
Service Historique de la Défense.

for the Germans. Over the next few months, the Gestapo arrested and imprisoned nineteen network members, including Boris Vildé and Yvonne Oddon. Paul Rivet, the museum director and network organizer, managed to escape. He fled to Colombia, where he had friends from anthropological research projects, and then to Mexico. Elisabeth de La Bourdonnaye was not so lucky. She was arrested and taken to the prison on rue du Cherche-Midi.

Her daughter Nicole knocked on Debré's door early the morning of March 23 to tell him. Stunned, he went on his scheduled visits to private patients, and then stopped at Elisabeth's apartment. Two of her three daughters, ages nineteen to twenty-two, were there. He was consumed by worry. "As one is with a gravely ill person, the heart clenched, the hope, the fear, the obsession, the feeling of life without her . . ." he wrote in his journal.[11] With Elisabeth's arrest, he seemed to be revisiting the terrible hours of his wife's death. It wasn't until several days later that they learned she was charged with having hosted at her apartment a supposed conspirator against the German Army. They also discovered that Albert Gaveau, the traitor who brought the network down, had wormed his way into serving as Boris Vildé's main assistant. He knew far more than he should have.

Debré began calling everyone he knew, looking for a lawyer to represent Elisabeth, suggesting fictional certificates to poor health, searching for a way to get her out. She was in prison, and he was tortured by his fear for her. "My love for her becomes crazy at times, with chagrin, anguish, remorse," he noted two days after her arrest.[12] He could not bring himself to walk past the prison, and told himself that she surely would have done so if their cases were reversed. He couldn't sleep. He heard her voice in his thoughts, telling him to cheer up. Then, at the end of April, a month after her arrest, he received a reassuring letter, full of love, from her. It helped. Her children were allowed to visit her briefly in prison in May. Then things tightened up, and there were only scribbled bits of notes, some written in blood, that she smuggled out of prison in the weekly exchange of laundry.[13] Elisabeth sometimes spoke of brutality and harsh conditions, but more often of keeping spirits up. "Surrounded by heroine hostages, sentenced to death; marvelous morale," she wrote.[14] As another month passed, however, Debré's spirits sank slowly into despair.

In April, Debré learned that Elisabeth had been taken to the Hôpital de La Pitié for treatment. He didn't know why: could old tuberculosis lesions be acting up? It gave him an idea. He bloodied a spot on a handkerchief and doused it with some TB bacilli, and sneaked into the hospital to the area where prisoners were kept. He had heard that sometimes patient-prisoners could be seen getting some air. If he could get the handkerchief to her, perhaps she would be released from prison for "treatment." He paced for hours, but no one emerged. Then he heard she was returned to the prison. On her side, Elisabeth's sister tried to use a family connection to German nobility, but that didn't work either. "Above all we counted on the prisoner herself, on her courage, her cool head and her intelligence, to obtain her liberation," Debré wrote.[15]

It wasn't until mid-August that Elisabeth was released on parole; the trial would not be held until January 1942. Debré was recovering from a minor surgery at the time, and he felt her return as a healing balm. "Admiration is not a strong enough word," he wrote in his journal on August 13. "I listen, breathing in her thoughts and words."

But on August 21, a Resistance agent shot and killed a German soldier at Paris's Barbes-Rochechouart Metro station, in revenge for the shooting death of another Resistance fighter. It was the first assassination of a German soldier in Occupied France. In response, the German military command in Berlin ordered that one hundred French prisoners be shot as hostages. Would Elisabeth be caught in the backlash? The nation braced to see how far the Germans would go.

Dr. Robert Merle d'Aubigné, an orthopedic surgeon, had a meeting set up for the following day with a Resistance contact, who told him right away that the Metro shooter was one of theirs, and he had been wounded. Could the doctor help? Merle d'Aubigné agreed, and followed instructions for a second rendezvous, where a young woman took him to the cellar of a house in the Thirteenth Arrondissement of Paris. The young man had a bullet entry wound at the base of his neck, but no exit wound. The bullet could have stopped against his spine, or his carotid artery, either option a dangerous one. Only an X-ray would tell. Merle d'Aubigné arranged an appointment at the Protestant Deaconess Hospital, where he often worked, for 6 p.m., when most of the staff would be attending religious services. Only the nurse who handled the X-rays would know. At 6 p.m., he and the nurse waited. And waited. An hour later, they gave up. No one showed up, no message was sent. The next day he met his contact briefly and heard that the young man had been arrested on his way to the clinic. They expected he would be shot.

A few weeks later, a young woman turned up in Merle d'Aubigné's waiting room and said the fellow had escaped and was at her house, still needing medical care. "While she spoke, I was thinking: I don't know this woman. She could be an agent for the Gestapo," he wrote in a memoir. "I responded: 'I don't remember any such call. You must be mistaken.'"[16] She nodded and said she could see that he was careful. She stood up, placing her hands on his desk, and then left. Merle d'Aubigné found a Metro ticket on his desk, with five names written on it. He set up a meeting with his colleague Dr. Raymond Leibovici, who had been forced from practice under the anti-Jewish statutes and was working with the Resistance. Leibovici assured him he had done the right thing to send the woman off. Merle d'Aubigné handed him the Metro ticket. "*Merde!* It's him!"[17] Leibovici said he knew two of the names, but only one Resistance agent would know all of them. The injured man was Pierre Georges, better known by his Resistance *nom de guerre,* Colonel Fabien. He was a communist organizer and weapons expert who managed to escape the Gestapo's clutches time and again. He would go on to play key

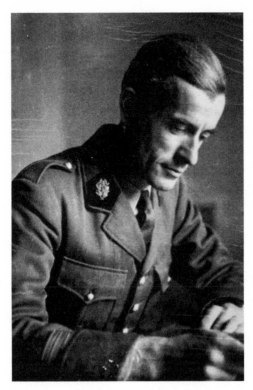

Dr. Robert Merle d'Aubigné, 1939.
Bibliothèque de l'Académie Nationale de Médecine.

roles in the Resistance, then joined the Free French Army, and died serving in eastern France in December 1944.

When the Germans were unable to put their hands on Pierre Georges, they designated ten hostages—down from the initial one hundred—to be shot in his stead. Among them was one of Elisabeth's cell neighbors in prison, Honoré d'Estienne d'Orves, a French naval captain who had begun setting up an intelligence network in Brittany for the Free French. Betrayed by an infiltrator, he was arrested in January 1941 and condemned to death after a trial in May, along with eight other members of his Nemrod network. On August 29, d'Estienne d'Orves was shot by firing squad, along with two others, at the Mont Valérien military fortress just west of Paris. They were the first Free French agents to be executed during the Occupation, and the fact that the Germans shot d'Estienne d'Orves—a conservative Catholic from a noble family—meant that no one was out of reach. It was a chilling sign to those who thought their social or religious identity would protect them. While still in prison, d'Estienne d'Orves helped his fellow prisoners to stay strong, leading discussions and holding conversations whispered through the cracks under their cell doors. Elisabeth helped smuggle out a letter for him, and Debré got it to his family. In June, d'Estienne d'Orves was moved to Fresnes Prison. In a last letter to his sister, written on the eve of his execution, he wrote: "No one should dream of avenging me. I desire only that peace and greatness be returned to France. Tell them all that I die for her, for her complete freedom, and that I hope my sacrifice will serve her."[18] Steeped in fury and sorrow at his execution, Elisabeth went to pay her respects at his tomb.

Debré had returned to Necker-Enfants Malades Hospital practice, but only as adviser to non-Jewish doctors responsible for patient care. When he was excluded, Pasteur Vallery-Radot had pushed all of his high-level contacts to get Debré exempted from the anti-Jewish statutes, and Debré was grateful. He had written in his journal: "PVR has all my admiration for his character, his courage, his clarity and his loyalty."[19] Then in September 1941, the chief of pediatrics at Necker-Enfants Malades Hospital announced his retirement, a position Debré had been in line to take before the Occupation. He saw no reason not to apply for it now. In the required vote by the council of medical faculty, Debré was approved unanimously, a rare event in that sharply competitive arena of medicine. "This is the greatest honor of my life," he told the council. "It is the honor of the faculty," they responded.[20] The right-wing press howled its disapproval. Necker-Enfants Malades in 1802 had become the first hospital in the world to focus solely on children. While he was not the first pediatrician in France, Debré is widely seen today as the pivotal doctor who focused medicine specifically on children, creating a specialization of their care. When a new hospital was built in northeastern Paris that merged the old Herold and Bretonneau Hospital services, the result, inaugurated in 1988, was named Robert Debré Hospital. He became a key figure of French medical history, his contributions reshaping the medical profession in many ways (see the Epilogue). If Vichy and the Nazis had had their way, he would not have survived the war.

Elisabeth, as soon as she was free, went right back to saving people in trouble. The government conducted the first round-up of Jews on May 14, 1941, by issuing an official notification requiring foreigners, mostly Poles, to appear for verification of their immigration papers. Instead, more than 3,700 Jewish men were taken into custody and placed in detention camps; they were later transported to the Auschwitz death camp. A second round-up in Paris on August 20, 1941, sent more than 4,200 Jews—French and foreign—to the newly opened internment camp at Drancy, a northern suburb of Paris. The pace of arrests was accelerating, and as French Jews as well as foreigners were being taken prisoner, they sought desperately to hide their children from the authorities. Through a connection at Rothschild Hospital, Elisabeth took in a few children at a time in her apartment, got them back on their feet, fed, cleaned, dressed in new clothes. She and Robert found farm families to host them in the Loire Valley, near Debré's country home at Vernou. A nurse from Rothschild Hospital escorted the children on the train trip south. They told the farmers they were Flemish refugee children. Debré wrote that he didn't think the farmers believed him, but there never was a single denunciation. Debré and Elisabeth made false identity cards and ration tickets for the children before sending them south.

"Never, I believe, did we create so many fake illnesses, nor had we ever signed so many false certificates to avoid this or that trouble with the police . . . ," Debré wrote in his memoir. "We were helped not only by the complicity of our colleagues—radiologists and laboratory directors—but also by certain civil servants, including those in the police. My laboratory at Enfants Malades [Hospital] was far from the only one to distinguish itself as a fabricator of false papers."[21]

In January 1942, Elisabeth returned to the prison to stand trial. The president of the German Military Tribunal, Colonel Ernst Roskothen, asked her if she had known that her houseguest the year before, Léon-Maurice Nordmann, was Jewish. "In France we don't pay attention to that," she replied. Debré wrote that he was as impressed by her answer as Roskothen was surprised.[22] She was sentenced to four months in prison, released upon time served. She could walk away, but the fate of her companions extinguished any happiness in it. Of the Musée de l'Homme group members put on trial, seven men were condemned to death (including Boris Vildé), three women (including Yvonne Oddon) were sentenced to deportation to German labor camps, two women were sentenced to prison in Germany, and five other men and women were acquitted. Vildé, Nordmann, and the five others given a death sentence were taken to Mont Valérian outside Paris on February 23 and lined up, paper squares pinned to their coats to mark the target of their hearts for the firing squad. Vildé asked to be shot last, to carry the burden of witnessing the worst for his friends, and he was.

Robert and Elisabeth had no illusions, then, about the potential consequences of their actions. Yet they felt compelled to act, to carry on the fight for those who no longer could do so. And for all the people helped by false identity papers and sheltered children, Debré's particular skills as a doctor were not being put to use. PVR and Milliez, similarly frustrated, consulted with Debré. As individuals, the doctors had been called upon occasionally to treat an injured Resistance fighter or to provide a medical certificate that kept a prisoner of-war from returning to camp. Could they put together a more systematic organization and keep it secret?

They called in four other trusted colleagues: Robert Merle d'Aubigné, Thérèse Bertrand-Fontaine, Clovis Vincent, and Paul Funck-Brentano. Together, they formed the Resistance Health Service (*Service de Santé de la Résistance*) in March 1942. Each of them brought medical expertise, hospital access, a wide range of contacts, and officially sanctioned mobility to the effort. They also had strong social authority, in carrying the responsibility of their patients' well-being. Most of all, they brought their individual conviction that working against the Occupation was not only the right thing to do, it was the sole course of action. They would do whatever they could. The seven doctors covered a spread of age, experience, and background. Robert Merle d'Aubigné, born in 1900, was the son of the Protestant pastor of Neuilly-sur-Seine, a parallel to Debré's in belonging to a religious minority in that posh riverside town. He had interned under Dr. Thérèse Bertrand-Fontaine and specialized in orthopedic surgery. He had met Robert Debré in 1932, when his newborn daughter was ill and Debré was called in to consult. The baby recovered, and he and Debré became friends.

Thèrese Bertrand-Fontaine became the first French woman to head a hospital department in the early 1930s, and the first female doctor elected to the National Academy of Medicine (she was the third woman elected, behind physicist Marie Curie and nutritionist Lucie Randoin). Born in Paris in 1895, Bertrand-Fontaine rose to her accomplishments on the foundation laid by two prior generations of French women doctors, each of whom had pushed the ceiling a little bit higher. It had not been easy for them, nor was it for her. She was not one to duck a challenge either.

Clovis Vincent, a neurologist, was a pioneer of neurosurgery along with Dr. Thierry de Martel. Together they had traveled to Peter Bent Brigham

Hospital in Boston to study under Dr. Harvey Cushing, the founder of neurosurgery who also had operated as a volunteer at the American Hospital of Paris during the Great War. Cushing returned to Paris to see them and, after watching Vincent operate, pronounced him among the finest neurosurgeons in the world. Vincent, sixty-two, was chief of neurology at Hôpital de La Pitié when the Germans took it over. German police officers interviewing staff asked: Would he promise not to treat Jews, Freemasons, or Communists? "I only treat patients," he replied tersely. He was transferred immediately over the wall, to the adjoining Hôpital Salpêtrière, not under German oversight.[23]

At forty-two, Paul Funck-Brentano was a practicing gynecologist at the Hôpital Broca. He later became allied with Robert Debré in the left-of-center National Front, and postwar, researched and published on the health consequences of deportation for women.

The group met for the first time at Robert Debré's apartment on rue de l'Université in March 1942. They assigned each other code names (PVR was Renoir, Debré was Flaubert), and Paul Milliez handed out cyanide pills, an ultimate option in case of arrest. They agreed to set up several projects: first, a laboratory to produce false medical certificates. Debré volunteered the basement of Necker Hospital, where he and Elisabeth had already set up a forgery shop, with the help of some members of the hospital staff, for the Jewish children they hid. Secondly, several stocks of basic medication and supplies needed to be gathered to be available to treat Resistance agents when needed. PVR suggested the Institut Pasteur for one stockpile. Thirdly, they needed to solicit the help of hospital personnel to hide those on the run, whether communists, Jews, or Allied airmen. Thus the Resistance Health Service was launched, and all agreed that its leader would be PVR. He was not the most senior, but he had the trust and respect of everyone in the room.

They would need to be careful. Jealous hearts and evil minds were everywhere, and the highly competitive field of medicine may have had more than its fair share. Even at the Institut Pasteur, one of the leading scientists, Ernest Fourneau, belonged to the collaborationist Franco-German Committee and worked closely with the Germans. The French police were flooded with denunciations, against neighbors, against rival merchants, against personal enemies but most especially, against Jews. Doctors were no exception.

Dr. André Cachera, secretary general of the Association of Former Doctors of Combat Corps, wrote to the government in July 1942 to insist that Dr. Raymond Leibovici be denied an exemption to practice, even if the Medical Order applied for one. "We favor maintaining the exclusion," Cachera wrote.[24] He received a warm reply from the Commission on Jewish Questions. Dr. Paul Guérin also wrote to Cachera from the Health Ministry to assure him that "the ever-growing number of demands for exemptions for exceptional services presented by the Medical Order Council has not escaped my vigilance."[25] He specifically named only Leibovici, French son of Romanian Jewish immigrants with an established leftist political profile, among the 250 doctors to be excluded. Leibovici was already a key Resistance operative by then.

Debré and Vincent had discussed regretfully a close friend of both who deliberately ended their relationship because he believed following Marshal Pétain was the correct path in the situation. Vichy's replacement of Work, Family, Nation for France's revolutionary motto of Liberty, Fraternity, Equality suited many people just fine. The doctors also heard, through friendly police sources, that both PVR and Debré had been denounced as anti-Vichy, and that another doctor had demanded that Debré be arrested. Not only were the doctors being denounced, but patients as well. "We knew that these informers had also denounced some poor refugees in our hospitals," Debré wrote.[26]

Antisemitic propaganda and acts ratcheted up intensely in 1941, becoming publicly visible in ways that they had not been before. The Nazis stoked the flames of hatred in France as they had in Germany. From September 1941 to January 1942, an exhibit was held in Paris entitled "The Jew and France" ("*Le Juif et la France*"). It had been organized by the Institute on the Study of Jewish Questions, an agency funded and directed by the German propaganda office. The *Paris Soir* newspaper announced the exhibit with entirely cynical enthusiasm: "It does not turn to any passion, any resentment, any hate. It stands to show, purely and simply, without commentary, the position of Jews in France, their tight grip on all the gears of command of political, literary and economic activity in France."[27] The exhibit attacked Jews in various professions, from cinema and art to business and politics, and in the medical section included a large panel with the photographs of thirteen Jewish doctors under the headline "Medicine: Quackery." It indicated that in 1940, there had been 1,853 Jewish doctors in Paris alone, 30 percent of the total number of doctors. The number was exactly double that reported in the government's own 1940 census.

Dr. Fernand Querrioux, a dermatologist who worked for the Institute

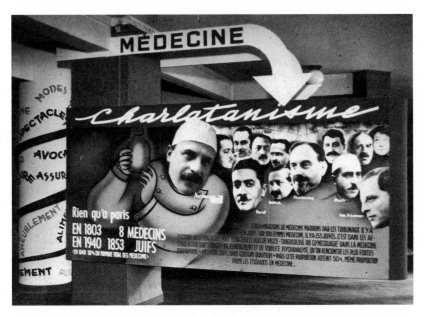

Poster denouncing doctors at a 1941 anti-Jewish exhibit in Paris.
Mémorial de la Shoah.

for the Study of Jewish Questions, had put together the medical component of the exhibit, an extension of his longtime ranting in the press against foreign and Jewish medical colleagues. *Le Matin* newspaper on September 24, 1941, noted that in a conference he gave at the exhibit, Querrioux had maintained a medical analogy of "the causes of the infection from which France nearly died. A pernicious anemia undermined our country and we were headed for a certain death." Beneath the brief article, the newspaper announced in large print: "All the French should go to the exhibit." It also pronounced, "They will learn that it is impossible for honest people to earn their living in a country where Jews are all powerful. And that is how it was in France." These were examples, aimed specifically at the medical community, of the Nazi narrative: that the Germans had rescued France from a dire fate. History offers a long and sad list of how a lie repeated often enough becomes a lie that is believed. And many French did believe the fascist propaganda of both *Le Matin* and *Paris Soir*. A reported 200,000 visitors paid three francs each to see the exhibit, which continued on to display in Bordeaux and Nancy. Louis-Ferdinand Destouches, the doctor better known as the author Céline, also attended the exhibit and complained to organizers that his works were not being sold as part of it. He had published a series of pamphlets criticizing Vichy for not being tough enough on Jews. He knew his market when he saw it.

From 1940 to 1944, the French press expressed one opinion: the Germans were fine, the Marshal was great, anyone who disagreed was an enemy of the state. In the newspapers' vocabulary, Resistance agents, or those who acted against the Germans, were "terrorists." The press did not often publicize acts of resistance, except when they resulted in the execution by shooting of French hostages, as in August 1941. The government's ability to control the narrative was far simpler in a time not just before the internet and social media, but before television. That is why the Resistance tracts, framing events in counterperspective, were important. The first issue of *The French Doctor* broadsheet explained why its authors were publishing it. "We will fight with all our force against all forms of obscurantism and all forms of smothering of thought, from wherever they come. We will fight so that our country, so rich in traditions, regains the path of progress. We will fight against the national oppression, for freedom and for the independence of France."[28]

By the time those words were in print, one of the paper's founders, Dr. Maurice Ténine, had been arrested. His publishing partner, Dr. Jean-Claude Bauer, was taken a year later. Both were executed by firing squad. The newsletter, picked up by dedicated colleagues, continued to be published through the Occupation, pushing back against government propaganda. Dr. Querrioux was noted in the very first issue as a front man for Vichy, a devoted follower of Hitler, and a physician who blackmailed and coerced his patients. "Mr. Querrioux is a dishonest doctor, a corrupt politician, and he is exactly characteristic of a man of the 'National Revolution,'" the paper said.[29]

Querrioux explained in an article in *Le Matin* on September 15, 1941, no doubt timed for the antisemitic exhibit, why doctors were so important.

"The doctor penetrates into the family existence, into the household secrets, into individual intimacy; over the course of a career that is, most often, a veritable apostolate, the doctor receives the most delicate confidences, he often has to treat the morale as well as the body of his patients."[30] Querrioux continued into his trademark rancorous racism, but he was correct in the idea that doctors had special entry into society. For the doctors in the Resistance Health Service, however, that privilege would be put toward saving their fellow citizens, and along with them, their nation.

4

RESISTANCE SPREADS ROOTS

While the Resistance Health Service organized as a medical assistance group, other doctors also created cells aimed at gathering intelligence and transmitting it to London, at carrying out sabotage operations, and at helping downed Allied airmen escape from Occupied territory. One of the largest groups, founded in early 1941 by three doctors, called itself Vengeance, and went to work with that in mind.

Dr. Victor Dupont had only been home from prisoner-of-war camp for two weeks, just through the Christmas holidays of 1940, when he started organizing a resistance group. He was thirty-six years old, married, and the father of two young children, and he practiced at Salpêtrière Hospital. While in the military prison camp at Melun, Dupont had gotten to know some intelligence officers in the French Army, who had subsequently escaped and were now working with the Vichy government in the Unoccupied Zone. Despite the much-publicized handshake between Marshal Pétain and Adolf Hitler at Montoire in October 1940, many French military and intelligence officers still believed Pétain was simply buying time, and the Germans would be thrown out of France soon enough. They invested in the so-called "double game" of cooperating with the Germans in public and hoping for their defeat in private.

Another group of French Army officers declined to participate in this waltz of hypocrisy. General Charles de Gaulle, politically astute, stubbornly patriotic, and willfully imposing, escaped the mayhem of France's collapse, arriving in London on June 17, 1940. The following day he delivered a four-minute speech on BBC Radio that changed the course of the war. France could fall back on its empire and its allies to continue the war, he said, and called on French military men to join him in London to fight on: "Whatever happens, the flame of French resistance must not be extinguished and will not be extinguished." De Gaulle and his partisans became known as "the Free French," in contrast to those in the metropole. Taking the double-barred Lorraine cross as their symbol, they drew their first adherents from French troops who had been deployed abroad when France surrendered.

From Vichy, meanwhile, the intelligence officers maintained secret contact with the Free French in London and with their counterparts in the newly created British Special Operations Executive (SOE). Dr. Dupont wanted to help them by providing information on German movements and actions around Paris. He recruited two fellow doctors—François Wetterwald and Raymond Chanel—whom he knew well and trusted, and they in turn began bringing in medical students, friends, and workers, especially those in the national communications and railway companies. Taking Vengeance as the group's name, they started watching and noting what they saw, and Dupont sent it on to London, secretly, via the intelligence bureau in Vichy.[1]

For the first year, from January until the end of 1941, Dupont traveled to Vichy once a month to report to his intelligence contacts. By early 1942, it was safer for them to send couriers to Paris to pick up the information. The Vengeance network had grown rapidly, expanding to include an operations section to carry out sabotage, as well as escape-and-evasion lines through the towns of Nevers and Angoulême, both along the demarcation line that split France into Occupied and Unoccupied zones. Dr. Raymond Chanel, an ear-nose-and-throat specialist with a practice in Nevers, oversaw the escape routes used by French former POWs, by Resistance agents whose identities and actions had been discovered, and by Allied airmen who had parachuted out or crash-landed in Occupied territory. The main route they used led through Pau, at the foot of the Pyrénées in southwest France, where they paid professional guides to take escapees across the mountains to Spain.

In the early years, expenses were reimbursed by the French intelligence service, but no agents were paid. Vengeance leaders met in Paris at the Caisse des Allocations Familiales, a government social services office, or in the presbytery of Sainte-Trinité Church in the Ninth Arrondissement, where the priest also helped create false identity papers for Resistance members and Allied aviators. By the end of 1942, Vengeance counted 150 operatives in the intelligence section and 50 in the action section. That expansion coincided with an acceleration in the dynamic of the conflict, pushed first by the American entry into the war, then with the Allied invasion of Vichy-held North Africa. The United States had maintained a semblance of neutrality for the first two years of the war, although its moral and material support for the British and Free French was apparent. In November 1941, when the Germans demanded the removal of the Vichy armed forces commander in Algeria—General Maxime Weygand's relations with the US representatives there were too amicable for their taste—Washington began to shift gears.

"[As it] appears from this point of view to be the real beginning of the Axis move to control the colonies, it is believed that this is an appropriate time to consider a complete revision of American policy in regard thereto," Admiral William D. Leahy, US ambassador to Vichy, cabled to the State Department.[2] Britain and the United States had been discussing the strategy of using North Africa as a springboard for an invasion of Europe from the south: if the Germans took it over, that option would evaporate. Leahy's message underscored the sense that time was running out. Within weeks, on December 7, 1941, the Japanese bombing of Pearl Harbor and US territories in Asia pushed the United States full throttle into the war. There would be no more doubletalk diplomacy or smokescreens over military aid, though the American nation was still far from ready to fight. In Occupied France, the news brought a rising surge of optimism. In the First World War, the arrival of American troops in 1917 had saved the nation and brought humbling defeat to Germany. The French, in the bitterly cold winter of 1942, warmed their hopes around that memory. The ranks of the Resistance grew, as now it seemed that clandestine counteraction would bring tangible support to the fight for freedom. At the same time, Allied bombing raids increased over Occupied territory. Royal Air Force commanders hoped that an intensive bombing strategy would knock Germany out of the war, without the need for a massive ground invasion. With the growing number of air raids came more and more aviators shot down or parachuted out over France. Many of them needed medical attention.

Dr. Robert Merle d'Aubigné had an apartment and office on the quai Voltaire, across the river from the Louvre Museum, for his orthopedics practice. One day he found a young British man in his waiting room, speaking fluent French, who said he had hurt his knee.

"I injured myself on landing," he said. "My parachute took me over uneven ground."

"Your parachute?" Merle d'Aubigné responded, eyebrows raised.

"I am English, I work with the clandestine forces of the interior, organization, supplying arms, funds," he said.[3]

Merle d'Aubigné wrote in his memoir that he did not know how the man had found him or had known that he would be a safe person to go to. "I couldn't believe my ears," he wrote. He told the agent his knee needed surgery, and the man said he would have it taken care of in England.

"Do you go there often?" Merle d'Aubigné asked. The man explained that he had been in and out of France for six months and would return to England before long. Then he left. Two weeks later, Merle d'Aubigné received an anonymous note: the man had been arrested, he may have had your address on him, don't go home. Merle d'Aubigné stayed away for a week, but there was no sign of surveillance or inquiry, so he returned. He later heard that the man had been shot. He wrote that he was filled with admiration—and concern—for these young men who risked their lives with such casual courage. So when Robert Debré and Louis Pasteur Vallery-Radot asked him to join their Resistance Health Service, he didn't hesitate. Providing medical treatment seemed the least contribution he could make to the greater fight.

At a hospital one day, a nurse introduced a friend of hers, and left them alone. The woman immediately asked if he could come see a wounded American airman she had taken into her apartment. He wrote that he went with her to the Fourteenth Arrondissement and found a feverish young man with an infected broken elbow. Merle d'Aubigné asked what had happened. His plane had been shot down over Senlis, northeast of Paris, and the attacking German pilot had sprayed him with machine-gun fire as his parachute descended. He made his way to a farm, where the farmer's wife gave him a meal, civilian clothes, and took him by train and taxi to a Paris clinic where she knew a nurse. He was treated there, but two days later the clinic director decided it was too dangerous to keep him. So the nurse took him home. "What else could I do?" she asked.[4]

Merle d'Aubigné, noting in retrospect that at the time they did not have the simple solution of antibiotics, cleaned out the wound, put the elbow in a plaster cast, and gave the airman a blood transfusion to boost his immune system. All in the nurse's bedroom. A month later, the aviator was in good enough shape to be handed over to an escape line and sneaked out of France. "I later learned that after the war that he had returned to see his helpers: I believe he brought them an American medal," Merle d'Aubigné wrote. "They had certainly earned it."[5]

Merle d'Aubigné had already had some personal interaction with the forces they were up against. His wife, born Anna Gunzberg, was from a family of Russian Jews who had immigrated to France at the turn of the century. She was not religious, and thought Merle d'Aubigné's prominent Protestant profile would protect her. His ancestor, Théodore Agrippa d'Aubigné, was a famous poet and Protestant leader in the sixteenth-century wars of religion. Anna did not consider that she was in danger. Robert thought she was naïve.

The General Commission on Jewish Questions had issued a questionnaire in July 1941, first a short model that asked respondents to "swear on their honor" that they were not Jews.[6] The long form that followed asked seven questions about grandparents, parents, and spouse. By the end of July, the mayors of France were told to compile lists of all Jews who lived in their towns, or in the case of Paris, their arrondissements. In the fall, all persons on these lists had to get a new national identification card, stamped "Juif" or "Juive" according to gender. Anna Gunzberg had four Jewish grandparents. The Germans gave her a week to provide proof she was not a Jew.

In the meantime, Anna had moved to the Unoccupied Zone, but it would not be far enough from the grasp of the Germans. Merle d'Aubigné dropped everything to meet her on the Swiss border, hike with her through the Alps, and get her to safety. Her son from a previous marriage was studying in Switzerland at the time; she would live near him. With her settled, Merle d'Aubigné returned to Paris and got back to work. But Anna returned to Paris within months; she was lonely. And in the meantime, the rules on identification had tightened up even further. They would have to come up with something.

Merle d'Aubigné found a Russian artist to draw up four birth certificates of pseudo-tsarist vintage, covered in official stamps, on yellowed paper with deep folds. He noted ironically that they were clearly precious works of great art, given the price he had paid for them. They would be submitted as evidence that Anna Gunzberg was not a Jew. Merle d'Aubigné delivered them to the General Commission's headquarters; he was summoned to return a month later. He found the office sinister, those waiting in the reception area stiff with terror. He was called in to an office, where he was handed the certificates with a black line drawn across them, labeled "False." The

German police had examined them too closely. The commission representative asked if he knew Dr. George Montandon, the commission's expert on Jewish identity. "Go and see him. He is your only hope," the man said.[7]

Merle d'Aubigné was reluctant. Montandon was a Swiss medical doctor who had studied anthropology in France and considered himself a racial scientist. He had published a pamphlet, *How to Recognize a Jew,* in 1940 and was quoted widely in the antisemitic press on physical and cultural attributes that distinguish "races." Before the war, Montandon had worked at the Museum of Natural History with Paul Rivet, with whom he developed a deep rivalry. The writer Céline reported that Montandon would turn beet-red in "blusters of hate" when Rivet's name arose.[8] Montandon, like the Nazis, believed race was an identifiable biological attribute; Rivet considered that social and cultural aspects determined categories that were commonly referred to as "race." Even before the war, in March 1939, Montandon had given a conference (at the invitation of the notorious antisemite and fascist Louis Darquier de Pellepoix) on physical characteristics of Jewish people that were different from those of French people. Montandon was widely accused of antisemitism, which was not a problem for him. In 1941, for example, he protested vehemently to the government when Robert Debré was reinstated as professor at the Paris Medical School and as a hospital practitioner. "He speaks well, he teaches well, but the value and originality of his discoveries are null; they are pseudo-discoveries, cleverly presented as advances," Montandon wrote, in words that better described his own work than Debré's.[9]

In 1941 Montandon helped launch a newsletter titled *L'Ethnie française* (French Ethnicity), financed by the German Institute of Paris, and in each monthly issue wrote an article critical of Jews, while other articles praised French-German collaboration. That same year, the Germans proposed lending a German expert on racial identity to the General Commission on Jewish Questions in order to consider any appeals for identity exemptions. Commission director Xavier Vallat suggested Montandon take the position instead. Thus Montandon was not only the Germans' front man in their campaign against Jews; he was Vichy's pseudo-scientific façade for painting the French as Aryan. In articles and conferences, he explained that the northern French were of the Nordic race, the eastern were of the Alpine race, and the southern were of the Mediterranean race, all of which should be considered Aryan—and "races."

Merle d'Aubigné went to see him. If Montandon said Anna was Aryan, she would be safe. He was prepared to pay (again) for such a determination. Montandon's official fee was 400 FF, but he had a sliding scale upward where proof was lacking. One man recounted paying 50,000 FF through a lawyer to obtain a certificate saying that while his circumcision indicated he was Jewish, after a thorough examination Montandon found it was not the case. If someone couldn't pay, they were found to be Jewish after all. At one point, Montandon tried to get the Union Générale des Israélites de France (UGIF), the Jewish social protection agency, to pay his fees.

Merle d'Aubigné discovered that Montandon's obsession, apart from race, was circumcision. In their interview, Montandon asked first if Anna's brother was circumcised, to which Robert replied he did not know, and the brother was abroad. What about their sons? Anna had two sons from a previous marriage, both out of the country as well. Robert did not know. "My own son, I can tell you, is not circumcised," he said. Montandon looked at him. "What about you? Show me!"[10] Merle d'Aubigné wrote that his strong desire to punch Montandon in the face made it difficult to undo his pants, but he did, and passed the test. Submitting to the humiliation of an inspection, plus handing over a hefty fee in cash, got him a declaration that said Anna "may be considered as non-Jewish, for the time being." It was enough to get Anna an ID card without a Jewish stamp. Robert was as disgusted as he was relieved. The experience added to his determination to fight.

At the same time, he and the other doctors felt frustrated by the limits on their ability to act. Joining ranks with Robert Debré, PVR, Paul Milliez, and Thérèse Bertrand-Fontaine helped give Merle d'Aubigné a focus. They could combine efforts and resources, which multiplied their effectiveness. By mid-1942, their Resistance Health Service counted 120 doctors and medical students, organized in units of five persons known only to one leader. Other doctors also were involved in different resistance groups. Dr. Robert Monod, a thoracic surgeon who specialized in tuberculosis, hid operatives in his clinic in the Paris suburb of Franconville. He headed the medical service for the Resistance group *Défense de la France*. Monod's wife and son Claude, both also doctors, were active resistance agents as well. In 1944, Claude Monod took charge of the guerrillas in southeastern France.

The Paris doctors, all working in and out of the same hospitals, knew one another, but there seems to have been little interaction of Resistance activity before 1943. Paul Milliez explained in his memoir: "Sometimes a good friend of whom you were sure then revealed himself a coward, or won over to the cause of the Germans, or more frequently Vichy. Others—and they were many—were already involved up to their teeth in a network, avoiding us like the plague, and of course didn't say a word."[11]

In June 1942, the authorities began requiring Jews to sew a yellow star to their clothing, under threat of arrest if they failed to do so. Robert Debré, however, simply refused. It was a colleague at the Academy of Medicine who reported him to the police, after he attended a meeting without the Star of David on his suit. An inspector went to his home. "Interrogated, the subject declared himself to be Jewish and to not wear the star, after having been exempted from all the interdictions of the statute on Jews [. . .]. According to his statements, the occupying authorities have always made an exception for him. Recently after his telephone was cut off following a denunciation, the occupying authorities had it reinstalled immediately."[12]

Despite—or perhaps because of—Debré's stature and popularity, he was regularly targeted by antisemitic colleagues. By August 1943, some 26,000 Jews in the Paris region were officially registered as wearing the yellow star.[13] Refusing to wear it carried great risk. A colleague of Debré's at Necker Hospital, Dr. René Bloch, was arrested for pinning his WWI medals beside his yellow star. He was deported and died at Auschwitz. The police inspector's report continued:

> Professor Debré adds that he has presented himself several times in German offices without the star. These services know his identity on the one hand, but have always considered that he was not Jewish, according to the expression given in the decree of 5 January 1941. At the time wearing of the star was announced, the Préfecture of Police was queried, and he was told that he was in a special category by virtue of the decree. In the Medical Order, Professor Debré is not registered among the Jewish doctors; his case is considered distinct.[14]

The inspector concluded that Debré did not have a dispensation to not wear the star, but that "given the personality of Professor Debré, we are satisfied to confine our mission to investigating his case without citing an infraction."

A General Commission for Jewish Questions official reported in March 1943 to the German commander of the SD police, Heinz Röthke, that 205

Jewish doctors were authorized to practice in the Paris area. "Nonetheless, finding that figure excessive, I have asked today the Council of the Department of the Seine of the Medical Order to please furnish two lists." The first list would contain 108 names representing the 2 percent ceiling on Jewish practitioners; the second list would show those authorized to practice beyond the ceiling limit because of exceptions. Close examination of the doctors' military service will no doubt eliminate many on both lists, the official wrote. "Confident that you will confirm my point of view on this subject, I remain persuaded that total deportation will greatly simplify all these questions."[15]

As for the accuracy of the lists, Dr. Fernand Querrioux, the Gestapo's man in medicine, had assembled more than sixty-five lists of doctors, by neighborhood and arrondissement, who were supposedly Jewish. Dr. Sumner Jackson, of the American Hospital, would have been surprised to find himself on one of them.

After the Allies invaded North Africa in November 1942 and the Germans took over all of France, eliminating the Unoccupied Zone, the Vengeance network found itself with no connection to London. The intelligence officers in Vichy who had been network contacts had fled to join the Free French abroad. Dr. Dupont had to arrange with another Resistance group, *Ceux de la Libération,* to continue access to funding and communication. The group's contact with the Free French was Col. Frédéric-Henri Manhès, a former book editor and military commander, whom Dupont later would get to know well, at Buchenwald. London also took over financing for the network, through the Free French Bureau Centrale de Renseignement et d'Action (BCRA), in the amount of 200,000 to 250,000 FF a month. The money mostly was used to support about fifty agents who lived clandestinely, with no other source of income.[16]

At about the same time, Vengeance split formally into two groups, with Turma-Vengeance under Dupont handling intelligence, and a Corps-Franc (Shock Troops) under Dr. François Wetterwald organized in a military structure to carry out sabotage and prepare for an uprising. The Corps-Franc, founded in January 1943, began with one company of one hundred men and expanded rapidly to ten thousand men and women by June. Yet there was far more will to act than means to do so.

"We were often in difficulty and even in danger because of the almost continual penury of money we experienced," Wetterwald wrote in his 1946

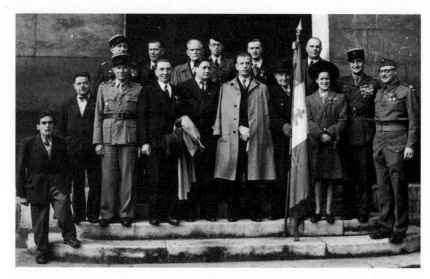

Agents of the Vengeance Resistance network, postwar. At center is Dr. Victor Dupont (raincoat draped over his shoulders) with Dr. François Wetterwald on his right. Marc Chantran Family Collection.

history of the Vengeance network.[17] "We were going to have to come up with something else."

Part of the reason for the spike in new members was that in February 1943, the German obligatory work program (Service du Travail Obligatoire, or STO) began requiring participation by all men between the ages of twenty-one and twenty-three, a group quickly enlarged to include up to fifty-year-olds. Many young men complied, but thousands of others went into hiding, joining Resistance cells in cities or guerrilla groups in the countryside. They had no means of support, neither ration cards to buy food legally nor income to buy on the black market.

One way to get out of being sent to work in a German factory was a medical certificate declaring a fellow unfit or ill. Doctors noted that they did not hand out disqualifications to anyone who asked for one. Without receiving a recommendation from a trusted friend, they feared being set up and arrested for fraud. Yet apparently enough doctors were lending a helping hand for the Vichy government to issue a warning in July 1943: "This manner of proceeding has done a great deal of damage, from the point of view of the clientele of the doctors of the Work Force, especially when the said certificates are issued by a local colleague. For this reason this manner of proceeding is forbidden in Germany."[18] Local doctors' assessments as to whether a patient was able to join the Work Force would no longer be accepted; they should only report a diagnosis, not a conclusion on a patient's fitness to work.

At the same time, the German authorities published threats of the direst sanctions against doctors who failed to turn in to police "terrorists" who came to them for treatment. One of the strongest tenets of French medicine is the doctor's adherence to secrecy; only the patient has the right to reveal health conditions or treatments. Doctors were infuriated when the Medical Order did not issue an immediate protest against what they saw as a clear violation of medical secrecy. "All doctors, before the silence of those who pretend to represent them before the nation, had to immediately choose between the threat of the occupier and their professional conscience," a medical resistance report to London noted. "All, or more precisely, almost all, because some have demonstrated the intention to obey without a murmur the German order if the occasion arose. These exceptions by their small number only underscore the irreproachable conduct of the majority of the medical corps."[19]

The summer of 1943 saw Vengeance's numbers double again, to twenty thousand men and women, and its funding from London rose to 2 million FF a month, about half of which went to Turma-Vengeance and half to the Corps-Franc. Sabotage operations primarily focused on trains and communications. For trains, a national railways (SNCF) engineer ran a week-long course in sabotage for 120 students, who then spread out across the country to test their skills. The list of delays they provoked in moving French goods and workers to Germany was long. In communications, one PTT (*Postes-Télégraphes-Téléphones*) worker managed to tap the Paris-Vichy telephone line, while another blew the Paris-Berlin telephone line by connecting it, to explosive effect, to a neighboring high-power electric line, via a kite with a copper-wire tail. The agent carrying out the connection was knocked unconscious by the powerful jolt. Then, in October 1943, Wetterwald organized an attack on the Germans' STO office on rue de Francs-Bourgeois in central Paris, destroying some one hundred thousand files on potential and truant workers. In another of their main operations, agents stole twelve German cars off the Champs-Elysées using a passkey, as well as a dozen German uniforms from public swimming pool dressing rooms. They also burglarized two Paris-area mayor's offices to steal ration cards.[20]

While overseeing the network, Dr. Wetterwald continued his medi-

Postwar Resistance identification card of Dr. François Wetterwald, a founder of the Vengeance network. Service Historique de la Défense.

cal practice. "It was great cover," he wrote. "The liaison agent brought the mail to the hospital and it was in the residents' library at the hospitals—Broussais, then at Salpêtrière—that I hid the archives."[21]

The Gestapo was on to Dupont by late 1942. Before they saw him, Dupont spotted the agents who came to arrest him at Salpêtrière Hospital. He told a colleague to send them to another end of the building, borrowed a coat, and slipped out the door. He warned his family to move, and went into hiding, staying with friends or in various apartments. He contacted Dr. Wetterwald, and asked him to take charge of Vengeance. Raymond Chanel had already been arrested in October 1942, imprisoned, and deported to the Mauthausen concentration camp.

Relations with *Ceux de la Libération* (CDLL) representatives, now more important than ever, became complicated by politics and personalities, the constant understory of conflict in the Resistance. Funding from London was arriving later and later, and in smaller amounts. It was coming through the CDLL network, now dwarfed by the ranks of Vengeance, yet still holding the purse strings. Dupont wanted to open a direct line of communication and supply with London. A rendezvous with an English agent was set up at the end of September 1943. Dupont hid in a false closet on a fishing boat to wait off the Brittany coast three times, but the English speedboat supposed to liaison with him never showed. On October 8, 1943, he returned to Paris. The next day, going to a clandestine meeting, he found the Gestapo waiting for him outside the Gare Montparnasse. One of his contacts had been arrested and turned, for money.[22]

At Gestapo headquarters in Paris, Dupont was interrogated and beaten, suffering a ruptured eardrum. His interrogator was a Belgian, Georges Delfanne, who told him flatly: "You played, you lost, now you pay." Dupont said later that he spoke at length, saying nothing of any use to the Gestapo. He noted in his postwar reports that no one in the network was arrested based on information he had given. An agent he was supposed to meet, Jean-Marie Charbonneaux, Vengeance's treasurer, had been shot and killed. The Gestapo showed Dupont a photograph of his body. Dupont was imprisoned at Fresnes, then at the Compiègne internment camp, and deported to Buchenwald in January 1944. But the leadership of Vengeance had been set up to continue operations despite the loss of individuals. Wetterwald ran it until he also was arrested in January 1944, deported to Mauthausen concentration camp in April. Then another member stepped up to lead.

Both Dupont and Wetterwald were nominated to the elite ranks of the Order of Liberation (*Ordre de la Libération*) by army officers who worked with them in the Resistance. Explaining their contribution, the officers noted: "The bases were solidly planted and despite the hard hits the Gestapo struck on many occasions . . ., Vengeance remained in place to play a historically important role in the military action against the occupier before the liberation of the nation. Their successes and their losses, through the years of the Occupation, in their actions, at the executioner's post and in the camps offer perfect testimony."[23] Nonetheless, neither Dupont nor Wetterwald were among the thirty-six doctors named Compagnons. The Order of the Liberation, created by de Gaulle in 1940, inducted 1,032 men and six women, and then closed to new nominations in January 1946. It was a knighthood of the old school, loyal to its king.

Postwar, 30,000 individuals were reported to have worked for Vengeance. The toll on them was heavy: more than 500 died, either in operations, at arrest or during deportation, while nearly 1,000 agents were arrested between 1941 and 1945. Nearly every Resistance network was infiltrated by French traitors secretly working for the Germans; it was impossible to ferret them out. So while some doctors who were close friends trusted and relied on each other, they did not bring up the subject of resistance to colleagues whom they didn't know well.

"Unfortunately, there were as many networks of denunciation as there were networks of resistance," Dr. Alec Prochiantz, a young medical resident and member of Vengeance during the war, recalled in an interview in 1994.[24] Professional solidarity was not to be counted on. When Wetterwald was arrested in January 1944, Prochiantz took up a collection among hospital staffers to help support Wetterwald's mother, who had been left with little means. He recounted how one doctor refused to donate. "He said 'That will be without me. With a name like that, he is certainly Jewish. We will have trouble.'"[25]

Prochiantz's father was Armenian, and had left his mother, a Russian Jew, when Prochiantz was a toddler. Alec Prochiantz had worked his way through medical school, hiding his mother with a non-Jewish family after a friendly policeman warned that she was not safe. A fellow medical student and friend introduced him to members of the Vengeance network, and he helped occasionally by writing prescriptions or hiding patients in clinics. It was an introduction to what was to come. In September 1943, a British acquaintance who lived in the western Paris suburb of Triel-sur-Seine called Prochiantz.

"Alec, could you come to Triel, I have a great gift for you, but it is fragile, I don't want to go around with it," the man said.[26] The "gift" was an American pilot who had bailed out of his burning B-17 the 'Yankee Raider,' returning from its third bombing mission over Stuttgart for the 384th Bombing Group. Second Lt. James E. Armstrong, of Bradenton, Florida, had just turned twenty-two. Having jumped through a flaming escape hatch when he bailed, he had burned his face and hands, and sprained his ankle in a rough landing.[27]

Prochiantz and a friend went to Triel to verify that the man was in fact an aviator and not a Gestapo plant. They sent his information to be checked

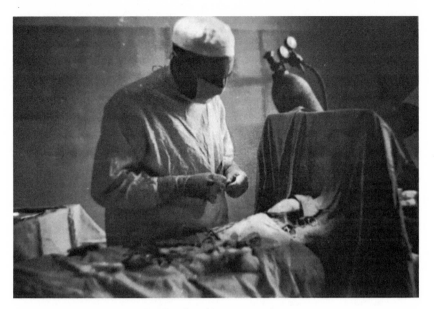

Dr. Alec Prochiantz operating.
Collection of Florence Prochiantz.

through London. It was confirmed, Armstrong was who he said he was. He had walked for three days, supplied by strangers along the way with food, civilian clothes, and even lessons from a farmer on how to walk like a French farmer and not, absolutely not, like an American soldier. They took him by train to Paris, and Prochiantz kept him, treating his burns, for two weeks in his apartment on the rue du Bac, in Paris' Seventh Arrondissement. Then he handed off Armstrong to Vengeance contacts in the northern suburb of Drancy, home of the dreaded internment camp. A Vengeance member ran a bistro in the town and hid people there. Armstrong was passed along the network to Brittany and eventually smuggled to England by boat on January 23, 1944. Of Armstrong's nine-member crew, five others also managed to evade and return to England, one was killed in the plane, and three were taken prisoner by the Germans. Vengeance leaders estimated in a postwar report that its escape line had helped move one thousand Allied aviators to safety.

Forty years after the war, Armstrong traveled to France to find and thank the dozens of French who had fed and sheltered him during his months of hiding, among them Dr. Prochiantz. In a memoir published in 2000, Armstrong wrote: "I shall never forget to give thanks for my French friends, who did not count the cost but risked much to reach out to me, a stranger."[28] He and Prochiantz later attended several reunions of airmen and helpers organized by the US Air Force Escape and Evasion Society (AFEES). By then, Armstrong was a retired Presbyterian minister living in south Georgia. Prochiantz was chief of pediatrics at the American Hospital of Paris. "[Helping] Armstrong gave me the impression that I really was in the Resistance," Prochiantz said later. "Everything we had, we gave to those guys."[29]

But there were lines Prochiantz was unwilling to cross. Some Vengeance members brought him an informant who had been shot in the chest by an agent, and asked him to help the man die. "I explained that I was ready to steal all the material they might need, but I would not use my profession to kill, even for a good cause," Prochiantz said.[30] He gave the man a shot of morphine, which helped him recover, and afterward the man repented of his betrayal and rejoined the Resistance. In February 1944, after several of his fellow Vengeance agents were arrested, Prochiantz went into hiding and then established a medical service with the rural guerrilla fighters called maquisards (see chapter 7).

While Vengeance was not primarily a medical resistance group, it did form a small medical section in August 1943. Joseph Heller, a Polish-born medical student from Clermont-Ferrand, was assigned with organizing cells of doctors, nurses, and others who could treat injured resistants and their families. Heller was arrested in May 1944 and deported to Buchenwald, where he found Dr. Dupont and joined him in working in a camp clinic. One of Heller's intelligence reports that was leaked to the Gestapo indicated that, contrary to international conventions on warfare, the Germans were using Salpêtrière Hospital to stock weapons and munitions. The doctors did not realize, in 1943, just how far beyond any rules the Nazis would go.

From its perspective in London, the BCRA could see each of the Resistance groups operating independently and sometimes less effectively that they might have. Thus in September 1943, the Free French sent a representative to pull together the various doctors into a *Comité Médical de la Résistance* (CMR) that could share resources and combine efforts. By the time the Resistance Medical Committee was formed, however, all the original Resistance Health Service doctors except Debré and Merle d'Aubigné had gone into hiding. London called them to meet with the BCRA representative, José Aboulker, a twenty-three-year-old medical student from Algiers. Accustomed to a certain show of deference from younger students, Merle d'Aubigné was taken a bit aback by Aboulker's confidence and direct manner. He gave them their assignments, not bothering to ask if they agreed with them. Merle d'Aubigné wrote in his memoir that he felt then the gathering strength of the Resistance.

"That's when I began to perceive the direction of the action that up to then, I had been pushed toward only through a visceral horror of missing out of a vital struggle for us, for the world," he wrote. "As insignificant as it might have appeared at times, absurd even, our action had not been in vain, our friends had not died for nothing, had not been tortured purely in loss. We represented—and de Gaulle incarnated for us for a long time already—the loyalty of our engagement to the pursuit of the war, the revenge of the shame of Munich, of the armistice, of the round-ups of the Vélodrôme d'Hiver, of the handshake at Montoire."[31]

Merle d'Aubigné noted that after the war, after having shown his intelligence, courage, and skill at command (and being named to the Order of Liberation), Aboulker applied, like any other student, for the medical school entrance exam. From a prominent Jewish Algerian family, Aboulker went on to become a neurosurgeon.

Within months of signing on with the CMR, both Merle d'Aubigné and Debré found the Gestapo at their doors. Merle d'Aubigné actually passed the agents on the stairs of his building, as they were headed to his apartment. He did not go home again. They came for Debré at his practice, and he managed to slip out a back door. He and Elisabeth de La Bourdonnaye went to stay with friends in a Paris suburb. From their clandestine shelters, the doctors did the work of the Resistance Medical Committee. Territory was split into a southern zone, overseen by Dr. Maurice Mayer in Lyon, and a northern zone, directed by Dr. Paul Milliez in Paris, who also served as treasurer. The Committee's assignment was to set up a medical service in contact with paramilitary and Resistance groups, so they knew who to count on when needed, and to provide treatment for bombing victims as the Allied air war intensified. Members also were asked to plan a medical service system for the liberation fight on the horizon. Among their tasks was the distribution of potassium permanganate for disinfecting water sources, if the Germans poisoned it in retreat. Merle d'Aubigné's particular assignment was to organize in the Paris suburbs mobile surgical teams, each consisting of a surgeon, a doctor, an anesthesiologist, a nurse and two assistants. They gathered stores of portable equipment that could be carried in two or three suitcases, stashed at someone's house until needed. They arranged for transport of patients by members of the Civil Defense or River Navigation units, both of which had passes to circulate after curfew.

Louis Pasteur Vallery-Radot had never hidden his support for de Gaulle and the Free French during the Occupation. It nearly cost him his freedom in 1942, when the British press ran an article about how he had evaded arrest by the Gestapo. They came looking for him again, and PVR and his wife went on the run. When the Resistance Medical Committee was formed, its members turned to him for leadership. There was a tremendous amount of work to be done, not simply treating wounded agents, but organizing medical supplies and distributing them to local clandestine "committees" across the country. PVR wrote in an article just after the war: "The point of these committees was to recruit doctors likely to give treatment to wounded Resistants and to act, in all circumstances, against the German authorities and the Vichy government. Wherever possible, the CMR was put in contact with civilian and military leaders of the Resistance. The CMR furnished these groups with material and subsidies needed for them to perform their patriotic duty."[32]

And along the way, PVR was always ready to enjoy himself. When a friend called in late December 1942 to let him know some Allied aviators were being sent to a safe house in Auteuil, not far from his apartment, he called Milliez to organize a party for them. "Americans!" he said. "What a wonderful thing on Christmas Day!"[33]

5

HARSH CONDITIONS, SLOW FAMINE

I f the solid foundation of good health is nutrition, by 1942 most of France was on very shaky ground. Food rationing, begun in 1940, had taken meat and milk from the market, butter and cheese from the shelves. The bulk of food production was sent to Germany or given to German troops occupying France. Those living in cities were worst hit, and they sought countryside connections for access to food. For Jews forced out of work, the situation quickly became critical. As early as August 1940, four canteens set up around Paris to feed Jewish residents were serving 1,500 meals a day.

At first, in 1940–41, the government cracked down on what it called black-market exploitation, explaining that the ration-card program aimed to even out the shortages among economic classes, so that those with more resources would not be able to simply buy their satisfaction. But by July 1942, the government had to cede to reality: people were starving. Police began to overlook food deliveries into Paris, and soon the government permitted "family packages" to be sent from the countryside to the cities. Workers' canteens were organized to provide a collective source of food. At the American Hospital of Paris, managers set up a pigsty in a garage and arranged for weekly deliveries of produce from a farm outside Paris to feed patients and staff. The research Institut de Biologie Physico-Chimique (formerly the Institut Edmond de Rothschild) in Paris's Fifth Arrondissement planted its grounds with vegetable crops, selling produce to local residents. In cities across northern France, people were desperate.

France had sunk into a state of "slow famine" by November 1942, according to Dr. Paul Le Noir, president of the Academy of Medicine and its Food Rationing Commission. Speaking for the medical profession, he launched a public appeal: "The Academy of Medicine, concerned about the progressive reduction in the nutritional value of rationed foodstuffs available to the population, and equally troubled that it is becoming increasingly difficult, if not almost impossible, for the less fortunate to meet their minimum nutritional needs, believes it is its urgent duty to alert the French government to the public health risks that a prolonged state of undernourishment can create."[1]

The severe lack of nutrition during the Occupation would have consequences for generations. Apart from famine edema, in which the body swells with excess liquid, and increased tuberculosis, doctors were finding stunted growth in children. By 1944, the lack of nutrition had cost children seven to eleven centimeters in height.[2] The medical community protested cautiously as a group, while individually, many doctors could not contain their ire. Dr. Charles Richet, a specialist in nutrition and digestion, was among the most vocal in the protests. Richet, sixty-one years old, son and namesake of a Nobel Prize laureate physician, was quoted by a medical student as shouting in his university lectures: "The Krauts are starving the French population!"[3] In February 1943, Richet gave a speech to the Academy of Medicine on the deleterious effects of a diet lacking all fats. A month later, he signed a dire announcement in the Bulletin of the Medical Order: "I affirm that ten million French in cities are suffering from slow famine: that two million of them are likely to succumb to hunger, whether indirectly from the spread of infectious diseases, or directly."[4]

Estimating people's fat intake at a quarter of what it was before the Occupation, Richet urged his fellow doctors to tell their patients to eat as much fat as they could find. (Fat is important in diets for helping vitamin absorption, among other roles. Today, doctors recommend that about 30 percent of daily calories should come from fat.) Even doctors who had been early Vichy supporters, such as Dr. Victor Balthazard, former dean of the Paris Medical School, were beginning to express alarm. Stung by the warnings from both the Academy of Medicine and the Medical Order, the government reacted through a statement from Marshal Pétain. He said he was aware of the problem and would ask the government to "examine the measures that may be taken to limit the serious risks that undernourishment of the French population may constitute for the future of the race."[5] Proposing a government study as solution has long been a way to avoid addressing a problem.

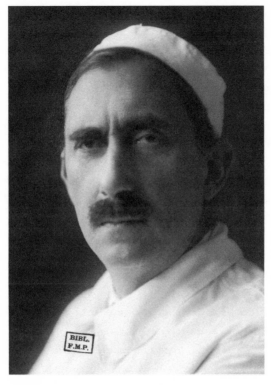

Dr. Charles Richet.
BIU Santé médecine—Université Paris Cité.

Food supplies in France continued to shrink, while shipments to Germany departed steadily.

When Richet was arrested in April 1943, friends assumed it was because of his protests over the food shortages. But the Gestapo interrogators were not interested in that; they wanted to know about his Resistance connections and operations. Richet had joined the Resistance group *Ceux de la Libération* in June 1942, and he directed its medical service. His six children and his wife—whom he met when they were both medical school residents—all were working in various Resistance groups. He wrote later that they never discussed it, and none knew what the other was doing. It was safer that way. When Richet and some fellow Resistance agents were held together at the Fresnes prison before questioning, they managed to put together a story that limited damage to the network. They learned eventually that their names had been found written on an uncoded list kept by one of the *Libération* network members who was arrested. In his memoir, Richet did not spare his disgust: the "imbecile" had "the intelligence of a sub-pen-pusher."[6] The man, whom Richet did not name, died at Buchenwald.

A report written in June 1943 and sent to London by the left-leaning National Front doctors noted that German biologists considered a daily intake of less than 1,600 calories as famine level, but imposed rationing on the French that meant 1,000 calories for the very poor, and 1,400 calories for those who benefited from other sources of food. The report cited a study that showed high-school students had lost up to six kilos (thirteen pounds) in the midst of their adolescent growth spurts; children were getting rampant infections and young women were not menstruating. Tuberculosis was showing a 30 percent increase in the young "in extremely rare forms of malignity."[7]

After the war, a study showed the rate of deaths from TB had risen by a third during the Occupation, due in part to contagion in prison camps, and had hit young men particularly hard. When the new Vichy health minister tried in March 1944 to downplay the increase of TB cases in order to continue sending men to work in Germany, doctors responded with outrage. The Medical Order Bulletin printed a reminder in its next issue "that they must obey their professional conscience and none other."[8] Between 1941 and 1943, 12 to 14 percent of all deaths were due to tuberculosis. (Tuberculosis remains one of the top ten killers in the world, according to the World Health Organization, but has dropped to an infinitesimal level in mortality rates in France.)

Aside from rising disease, lack of nutrition was severely damaging the health of all of the French, in ways that did not always show. "All body functions are affected: weight loss is just the most apparent, but more deeply, the blood, the bone, the respiratory passages . . . are altered, rendering the subject vulnerable to maladies that find them with no defenses," the National Front report said.[9]

Not only was food scarce, but medicine was in short supply. Many medical products could only be bought with ration tickets from February 1941 onward. From 1941 to 1942, the supply of basic medical elements such as bismuth (used to treat diarrhea and syphilis) and iodine salts (needed for thyroid function and fetal development) had been cut by 75 percent as supplies were diverted to Germany. This shortage was accompanied by a "disastrous" lack of medical tools made of rubber or tin (gloves, sponges, sterilizing pots), as well as baby bottles and nipples; vaccines for diphtheria and tetanus, obligatory for children, were hard to find. Doctors remarked they didn't even have enough soap to wash their hands between patients.

The Germans also were confiscating the nation's supply of insulin, forcing the French to limit insulin doses to diabetic children and pregnant women. In March 1944, José Aboulker (code name Trompette), the Free French envoy to the Medical Resistance Committee, wrote to London in a tone somewhere between frustration and fury. "I have no idea if you have received any of the *Eleven cables* I have sent you through different routes ... and above all, if you have received my request to send powdered insulin. Diabetics are dying by the thousands," he wrote. "For the past year, doctors have had the right to prescribe insulin to diabetics only when they've fallen into a coma."[10] In his report, Aboulker outlined the structure of the doctors' organization, pointed out the need to decentralize stocks of medication, and requested, with a touch of irony, that London send, along with sulfonamides and anti-diphtheria vaccines, medication to treat venereal disease, "in order to mitigate the consequences of the joys of liberation."[11]

The following month, Aboulker renewed his demand for insulin, noting that the two kilos of powder he was requesting weighed less than a machine gun, which London seemed able to drop into France by the ton. In his April report, he announced that the group had managed to acquire and hide two thousand medical kits around the country. How did they do it? "[We] kidnapped reserves accumulated by overly clever wholesalers and producers; recuperated army stocks overlooked by the Germans; in many cases retook from the enemy material they had stolen from us; diverted resources from youth camps to the Maquis [guerrillas], and, with our miserable budget of one million [FF], increased by some debts, went to the black market for bandages and painkillers from across the Swiss border."[12] He wrote that because they were acting illegally, they were able to accomplish what the government could not. "It is striking to note that clandestinity has allowed what the official administration could not do. Our illegality has the great strength of being conscious of its goals and the even greater strength of not being glued to routine and to act quickly and directly."[13]

Funding was essential. Until early 1943, expenses for the medical resistance were paid out of pocket—mostly the fairly deep pockets of PVR and other members—while the group repeatedly asked the BCRA in London to send cash. They had to pay for clinical services for treating wounded resistance agents, as well as for transportation and daily needs. Furthermore, their stockpiles of pharmaceutical material had cost some 250,000 FF. Financial support for the Resistance, primarily funded by the British and American governments, was growing. In March 1943, the Resistance reported receiving 800,000 FF, split between northern and southern zones, and noted that the budget had been increased for April and May to 4 million FF. In January 1944, the budget for all Resistance groups in France was reported at 129 million FF (nearly $450,000 at the black-market rate of exchange). The money was packed in stacks of cash and parachuted into rural France, along with supplies, food, clothing, and weapons, to Resistance agents.

The BCRA, having changed its name in 1944 to *Bureau de Renseignement et Actions à Londres* to distinguish it from the now active team based in Algiers, sent a memo of explanation on the method: "At the start of each moon, the B.R.A.L. will let delegates of the Action Committee know the schedule of expeditions, and in particular provisions for split or regional conveyances. Simultaneously, this schedule will be sent by telegram to delegates in the [drop] zones." In return, the Resistance groups were required to send an accounting of expenses in a form distributed to them in December 1943. They also were requested to send notice of any losses or missing amounts. A report in December 1943 noted 230,000 FF missing from a package of 1 million FF, for example.[14]

Naturally, there was competition between Resistance groups for access to funds; once the money was in hand, reasons for not sharing it were easily found. By October 1943, even the head office in London was starting to sound exasperated. "The need to establish financing for the Health Service in a direct manner must be imposed, for reasons of material organization as well as to assure an exact control," an unsigned report said.[15] It provided the example of having sent 10,000 FF to a southern-zone clinic to cover the cost of care for five injured resistance fighters, two of whom belonged to a communist group and three of whom were part of the rural guerrillas. "We would have to establish separate bills for the two groups, which is complicated and impracticable." The writer noted that establishing any verifiable control of spending was "illusory." London ended up dividing funds by region, leaving it to group leaders to distribute as needed, and account for as they could.

Providing health care, whether public or clandestine, was challenged by a lack of both food and medicine, a situation hospitals felt keenly and devised various means to resolve. But none of the Paris hospitals, requisitioned by the Germans or not, had the compounded difficulties of the Rothschild Hospital. Founded as a private charity institution in the nineteenth century by the wealthy Jewish banking family's foundation, the hospital counted 340 beds and included an orphanage and a rest home when the war began. With the Occupation, the Rothschilds' assets were confiscated, and foundation funds that supported the hospital were cut off. It was placed under the management of the Union Générale des Israelites de France (UGIF), an agency created by the Vichy government to act as administrative representative and to oversee social services for Jews. Then, in December 1941, the Préfecture for the Seine Department decided that any ill prisoners from the Drancy internment camp, or those who needed hospital attention after a Gestapo interrogation, would be sent to Rothschild. Robert Debré continued to serve on the hospital board of directors; he wrote that he was the only board member still in Paris by then.

When Drancy began sending prisoners to Rothschild, the hospital director asked Dr. Robert Worms to oversee the medical service for their ward. Worms, forty-two, an infectious disease specialist, had been excluded from public hospital practice by the anti-Jewish statutes. He took over two wards of 100 beds—quickly expanded to 240 beds—set aside for the prisoners. The prefectorial agreement put security in the hands of the police, and medical care in the hands of the doctors. The police patrolled the grounds and the halls of the hospital. At first, the doctors held their ground. "It was understood that the independence of the doctors would remain absolute, concerning the type of treatment as well as the length of the hospital stay," Worms wrote in a later report. "Contact continued between hospital doctors and the Préfecture medical services, but without any control in the strict sense of the word exercised by them."[16]

In early 1942, the Préfecture began increasing pressure to return patients to Drancy, whether or not they were in physical condition to withstand the miserable conditions of the camp. The Préfecture's chief medical officer, Dr. Jean Tisné, appeared harsh to the Rothschild personnel, ignoring Worms's pleas to allow chronically ill patients to remain at the hospital. "Then the prefectorial services on one hand, and Dr. Tisné on the other hand, multiplied their demands to me to return the largest number possible of patients to Drancy, telling me that a prolonged hospitalization risked to appear to the occupation authorities as a sign of excessive kindness and could have most serious consequences for the whole group of prisoners," Worms wrote.[17]

In his report, he described the Drancy police security detail—French, not German—as rough-handed and abusive with the patients. He considered it a small victory in February 1942 to have gotten an X-ray machine set up at the camp to screen prisoners for tuberculosis. Then, after the hospital saw four prisoner escape attempts, three of them successful, the police cracked down even harder on Rothschild. Patients were no longer permitted to leave their wards or to wear pajamas. "Patients in better shape had to walk around the ward draped in their bed linens," Worms wrote.[18]

The German SS command made two memorable visits to Rothschild. On April 4, 1942, SS Captain Theodor Dannecker, head of the German Jewish Affairs office (*Judenreferat*), visited the hospital to harangue and harass Jewish patients and staff. When a resident doctor approached, Dannecker kicked him in the shin. He ripped the bandage off one post-operative patient, shouting "A Jew doesn't need a stomach to travel!"[19] Dannecker demanded that 60 percent of patients be returned immediately to Drancy, and when the hospital director, Samy Halfon, protested, he also was arrested and interned at Compiègne camp. (He managed to escape and join a clandestine group of guerrillas.) Dr. Charles-Jean Odic, who worked at Rothschild until his arrest and deportation, wrote that Dannecker was "a howling madman incapable of even a glimpse of lucidity."[20]

Over the following year, doctors and nurses took increasing measures to dissimulate patients' conditions in order to keep them from returning to Drancy, to the extent of performing minor but unneeded surgeries to prolong the patient's stay in hospital. From Drancy, over the four years of the Occupation, more than 67,000 people were deported, most of them sent to Auschwitz. The hospital staff was aware of the deportations, but not of what awaited their patients at Auschwitz. "We thought that they would be submitted to a hard fate, but we did not know about the gas chambers, we did not know they were going to their deaths," Debré wrote after the war.[21]

The Rothschild Hospital sometimes offered the only hope for stepping

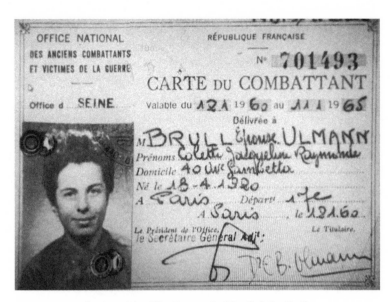

Postwar identification card of Dr. Colette Brull.
Service Historique de la Défense.

off that fatal path, and the staff did what they could, especially for children. Two hospital social workers set up a secret network to move children to safety; among their tactics was to provide non-Jewish names on birth certificates, and send the babies to live with families outside the city. Dr. Colette Brull, doing her medical residency at Rothschild as part of its Jewish staff quota, noted that the maternity department reported an unusually high number of stillborn births, but was in fact smuggling the babies out to shelter. Brull's father had been arrested and interned at Compiègne. "The only place I could act was here, at the hospital: delay the return of the ill to Drancy, as much as possible," she wrote. "Maybe I couldn't save my father, but I would save others."[22]

The social workers, Claire Heyman and Maria Errazuriz, kept Jewish children's names off the hospital registers when they could and sneaked them out of the hospital through the morgue, the only door that had no police guard. A priest gave the children baptismal certificates to provide cover identification. One night Heyman handed over to Dr. Brull a six-year-old girl and her three-year-old brother to take to a convent eight kilometers across town, on foot. With the girl by her side, Brull carried the boy through the dark and deserted streets, finally arriving at the assigned address, where a nun took the children in. "The fear came later, fed by the possibilities that came with reflection: fear of being surprised in the street, of getting the address wrong, fear that the children won't come along, that they'll start crying in the middle of the street," she wrote. "But none of that happened, so . . ."[23]

Instead, trouble came to Rothschild. At dawn on July 3, 1942, French police surrounded the hospital and rounded up all the prisoner-patients, even those who had to be carried out on stretchers. Dr. Worms noted that among them was a patient who had had stomach resection surgery the night before, along with others with severe cardiac conditions; some had clothes and others were taken in their pajamas. Worms arrived later that morning to an empty ward.

Two weeks later, on July 16 and 17, the police conducted their largest operation of the war, detaining more than thirteen thousand Jewish men, women, and children from a Paris neighborhood and dumping most of them, with neither food nor water, in the Vélodrome d'Hiver sports stadium. Both the number of arrests and the conditions of detention sparked a scandal among anti-Vichy activists. A half-dozen doctors volunteered to help the prisoners. Louis Pasteur Vallery-Radot and Elisabeth de La Bourdonnaye led a group to ask French Cardinal Emmanuel Suhard to intervene. Suhard wrote a letter of protest to Marshal Pétain, but, ever careful not to offend the occupiers, did not make it public. The prisoners eventually were deported to Auschwitz.

In February 1943, SS Captain Dannecker had issued a quota of prisoners to put on a deportation convoy from Drancy, but the police had fallen short in the number of arrests made. So he pointed them to Rothschild, with a list of foreign Jewish patients who had not been imprisoned previously. When even those patients did not fill the roster, he sent the police back to the hospital's rest home and orphanage, where police rounded up fifteen children for deportation. Dr. Brull watched them go, sick at heart, unable to stop it. One of the children, a seven-year-old girl, escaped by hiding under bedcovers. Fifty years later, after Brull gave a talk about the Occupation at Rothschild, a woman came up to her and said she was that girl. She had been handed over to the OSE (Oeuvre de Secours aux Enfants, a children's welfare agency), whose courageous workers led a group of thirty Jewish children on foot toward the Swiss border. The trip had been so rough, she told Brull, that only half of the group arrived safely in Switzerland.[24] At the Rothschild rest home, Dr. Odic wrote that in July 1943, the SS was not satisfied with an initial arrest of forty-one residents, all over sixty years old, and sent an officer back on the evening of weekly family visits. He managed to net another group of residents and visiting family members for a deportation convoy. "The German waited until every fruit was ripe, till every season was golden, till every action brought in its train a full load of ruin and suffering. He was determined to exploit the full power of suspense, to give to each wound a hitherto unknown depth," Odic wrote bitterly.[25]

Brull and most of the Rothschild medical staff considered it their duty to subvert the Nazis' insistence on returning patients to Drancy. "We falsified diagnoses, we exaggerated complications, invented tuberculoses," she wrote. "The SS were not doctors, after all. And what is more illegible than a lung X-ray, for a neophyte?"[26]

But the Germans did have French doctors working for them, the prefectorial medical officers, who visited Rothschild regularly to verify their reports. Brull wrote that she never forgave one of their doctors for having ordered two young sisters to return to Drancy. She and the rest of the staff had grown fond of the girls, hiding them for months in the hospital while their parents were imprisoned at Drancy. Both girls and their parents died in the gas chamber at Auschwitz. On another evening, Brull arrived to work and found the police covering two bodies in the courtyard. A mother had thrown herself and her newborn baby out of an upper window when the police came to take her back to the camp. Then one day, the Préfecture's doctor caught Brull encouraging an older woman patient, behind his back, to exaggerate her illness to avoid being returned to Drancy. The doctor ordered her brusquely to wait for him outside. She waited in anguish and trepidation until a colleague urged her to walk away and not come back. She left.

Dannecker's successor in June 1943 was Aloïs Brunner, an Austrian noted for his sinister half-smile and cold sadism. One doctor described Brunner as small in stature, nervous and slightly bowlegged. He came to Rothschild on July 5, 1943, to oversee another roundup of patients for deportation. Brunner informed the hospital staff that he was removing the police presence and that responsibility for any escapes would fall on them. His strategy, which he also employed at Drancy, was to turn the French staff and patients against each other. He left fifteen prisoner-patients in the hospital, and warned that if any one of them escaped, he would shoot forty-two hospital staff members. It made for terrifying tension. The following month, after a woman prisoner managed to slip away, the hospital director hurriedly wrote to the German authorities that he had hired private security guards to patrol at a cost of 40,000 FF a month, a figure that soon rose to 200,000 FF a month. Doctors later reported harsh interrogation of staff members following the escape, but no one was shot. Instead, the hospital director began requiring a medical resident to remain on duty every night, and if someone escaped, they would be held personally responsible. Doors and windows were nailed shut, and patients were no longer allowed to walk outside their ward. Dr. Alexandre Elbim described the situation in a postwar report: "The guards were given a red armband marked 'Rothschild Security Force.' Lacking guns, they got them another means of action: truncheons. Truncheons, bought by the Hospital, to use, if needed, against patients!"[27]

Then, in spring 1944, a hospital security chief was hired, a Frenchman known to be an informant for the Gestapo. He wrapped the entire building in barbed wire, rumored to be electrified, with a large sign forbidding anyone outside the grounds to speak to or communicate with a person inside, at risk of immediate internment. Dr. Elbim's report listed example after example of post-operative patients being dragged back to the internment camp, and squarely blamed hospital administrators and some of his fellow doctors, whom he described as more interested in obeying the Préfecture than in caring for patients.

After hospital director Samy Halfon was detained, Rothschild administrators were appointed by the government's General Commission on Jewish Questions. The administrators were not Jewish, and much of the hospital staff was not Jewish, but most of the doctors were. Both Dr. Worms and Dr. Elbim spoke highly of Halfon in their postwar reports. "The devotion he dedicated to the internees service, the courage and energy of his attitude, which ended up landing him in captivity, deserve nothing but praise," Worms wrote.[28] After the war, Halfon became a major film producer.

With the increased persecution of Jews in 1942, Dr. Léon Zadoc-Kahn, seventy-three, who had been chief medical officer of Rothschild Hospital since 1914, and his wife, Suzanne, went into hiding in a Paris suburb. They were denounced, arrested, and deported to Auschwitz; they did not survive. He and his wife had stayed in France despite early offers from his cousin, Eugene Meyer, the American owner of the *Washington Post,* to help them resettle in the United States, because they were devastated by the 1940 suicide of their son. Cardiologist Bertrand Zadoc-Kahn, who wrote that he could not live under the Nazis, took the same fatal step as did surgeon Thierry de Martel.[29]

Like Colette Brull and Léon Zadoc-Kahn, many of the Jewish doctors at Rothschild eventually went into hiding. Some went underground and joined the Resistance, while others, including Robert Worms, escaped France to join the Free French forces in North Africa. Worms served as a military doctor in the First Army and later on the command staff of General de Lattre.

6

PERSECUTION INTENSIFIES

The Drancy camp that received the first roundup of five thousand Jewish men on August 20, 1941, was an unfinished concrete public-housing complex, unfurnished, unequipped, and unsupplied with food. The Préfecture of the Seine was in charge, but the police saw their mission as maintaining prisoners' security, not their survival. The Préfect wrote to the Interior Ministry that the Germans had bedding and cooking material in the camp, but would not provide it for the prisoners, and the Préfecture had no budget for supplying and feeding such a number of people. The police had to go to prisoners' homes to collect their ration tickets in order to buy food for them. It wasn't until a week later, on August 27, that the German and French authorities responsible for the camp met to discuss who was going to take care of the prisoners. While they parsed out administrative duties, the ill got sicker and the hungry sank into starvation. Wrenched from their homes at dawn, many had nothing more than the clothes on their backs—often, pajamas.

The Préfecture's Dr. Jean Tisné was asked to set up an infirmary in the camp, and he quickly enlisted the help of Jewish doctors who had been arrested. He also invited the head German Wehrmacht (Army) doctor to visit the camp, and following his September 5 inspection, some 800 chronically ill prisoners were released. Tisné reported to him a list of another 250 prisoners whose conditions could not be treated in the camp: those with tuberculosis, cardiac disease, and syphilis, among others. "It appears impossible to organize at Drancy itself a medical and hospital service sufficient to assure these patients a minimum of indispensable care," Tisné wrote. Given that his instructions were to keep releases to a strict limit, he wrote: "It is important for me to know, in order to conform to it, the point of view of the German authorities on this subject."[1]

He also named four areas the camp direly needed to improve: the showers weren't working; there was no disinfection unit for vermin; there was no bedding for the prisoners, who were sleeping on raw concrete floors, and lastly but most importantly, they needed more food. "Without an increase in the nutritional serving by one means or another, there is every reason to fear the onset of high morbidity and mortality in the coming months," he wrote.[2] He urged the authorities to allow the prisoners to receive food packages from their families. SS Captain Dannecker refused.

By October, a camp food service had been set up, providing "a ration completely insufficient in number of calories (about 1,000 instead of the 2,400 theoretically needed) and poorly balanced because composed almost exclusively of green vegetables," Tisné wrote in a later report.[3] In fact, green vegetables were nowhere to be found, except on a theoretical menu imagined by the Préfecture that listed servings of meat and broccoli twice a week, along with potatoes and turnips. The harsh reality was a thin soup provided to prisoners twice a day. In late October and early November 1941, following subsequent visits by the German Army doctor, some 1,200 prisoners were released from the camp because of severe health problems, most of them due to starvation. The SS then was forced to allow food packages to be sent by families and social service agencies. But Dannecker, who had been in Berlin for several weeks, returned and put a halt to all further liberations, including that of a group set to be released the following day.

Provisions for hygiene also were lacking. Tisné noted in early 1942 that the camp's sanitary provisions remained entirely inadequate. There were sixty toilets for a population of nearly four thousand. "In case of an epidemic of diarrhea, such as occurred in November, the situation was lamentable," he wrote.[4]

The camp infirmary included five rooms with fifteen beds each, a small pharmacy, and Tisné's office and consulting room. He wrote that he oversaw fifteen Jewish doctor-prisoners, who were allowed to live together in the few apartments with bathrooms and kitchens. Among them was Dr. Samuel Steinberg, arrested by police in Neuilly-sur-Seine on August 21, 1941, while en route to visit an ill patient at home. Steinberg served as chief camp doctor from October 1941 to June 1942, when he was deported to Auschwitz. One of the few survivors of the extermination camp, Steinberg gave a lengthy report to the French government's *Service de Recherche de Crimes de Guerre Ennemis* (Research Service into Enemy War Crimes) upon his return to Paris.[5] The prisoners at Drancy, he said, initially served as hostages against attacks on German soldiers in Occupied France. "When they were faced with Resistance acts, they drew from the hostages and shot them," he said, noting that forty-three prisoners were executed as hostages in December 1941. At the top of the German lists were prisoners the Préfecture had identified as Communist Party or union members.

Then in 1942, deportation began sending a steady stream of prisoners to concentration camps in Germany. One day in June, Steinberg argued with Captain Dannecker about whether an infirmary patient was in condition to be transported, and Dannecker replied that he could join him and continue treatment on the way. Steinberg and the patient were packed into a cattle car with more than one thousand others, with no food or water, for the long and hellish ride from Drancy to Auschwitz. The first thousand prisoners were deported from Drancy on March 27, 1942, not knowing where they were going or what would happen to them. The camp's role shifted from internment to triage, with the pace of deportation convoys accelerating from one a week in June to four or more a week through the summer. Nearly thirty thousand prisoners were deported by the time the convoys paused for the winter of 1943. Quotas for deportation were set by the German command, and the French police were sent to arrest foreign and French Jews, who were kept in the squalor of Drancy until their names were put on a list.

In June 1943, SS Captain Aloïs Brunner took charge of Drancy. He had recently directed the deportation of 44,000 Jews from Salonika, Greece, and previous to that, 43,000 Jews from his native Austria. Under his command, entire families were arrested for deportation, and Drancy became the sordid home of men, women, and children. Brunner also removed the prefectorial administration (while keeping the gendarme guards) and put the prisoners in change of their own security, food, supplies, and maintenance. He named a French prisoner "commandant" of the camp, threatening dire measures of retaliation for any escapes.

Dr. Abraham Drucker, like Steinberg born in Romania and naturalized French, also found himself providing medical care for his fellow prisoners in the camp infirmary. Drucker, thirty-nine, had retaken his medical studies in France, as per the law, and in 1936 passed his exams. But as an immigrant, he was blocked from practicing medicine by the ever-tightening restrictions.

He worked in a tuberculosis sanatorium near Vire, Normandy, until his arrest and imprisonment in April 1942. The Germans accused him of being Jewish, of being a Resistance agent, and of being an Anglophile, and it was unclear which was the greater crime, in their eyes. He spent his first year of imprisonment at the internment camp in Compiègne, then in May 1943 was transferred to Drancy. When Steinberg was deported, he became the chief medical officer of a team that now numbered nearly thirty prisoner-doctors.

Drucker was made to accompany Brunner to Rothschild Hospital in July, along with two other Drancy doctors, to select patients to return to the camp. It was a losing gambit from any angle. If they took the most fragile patients, they would be least likely to be deported, but might not withstand the conditions at the camp. If they took the strongest patients, they would be on the next convoy east. "The most delicate moral problems arose. Those for Drancy had to be chosen without taking into account one's feelings, nor solicitations, nor imperative considerations that might be dictated by compelling ties or pity," wrote Dr. Charles-Jean Odic.[6] Odic recounted that one of the prisoner-doctors found his mother among the Rothschild patients. He had not seen her since his arrest months before. His first idea was to take her back to Drancy with him so they could be together. His companions observed gently that she was one of the most elderly patients, and unlikely to survive. He realized with sharp sorrow that he had to leave her behind.

In a postwar report, Drucker wrote that SS administrators made the rounds of the infirmary to judge with entirely unqualified eyes who was strong enough to deport. Contagious disease, such as tuberculosis and scabies, could disqualify a prisoner from deportation. Drucker was required to draw up lists of those who were contagious, and because the Préfecture doctor and nurses were observing, it was not easy to fake diagnoses. Sometimes Drucker and his fellow doctors were able to save a prisoner from deportation, but if they were caught in a medical manipulation, they would find themselves in an eastbound cattle car. "Delivered to the whim of these brutes, our existence wavered between anguish, terror, uncertainty and mystery," Drucker wrote. "No one knew where they were going or why they were going."[7]

There were rumors and suspicion. Prisoners who left Drancy were never heard from again; deportees were stripped of all possessions before boarding the train, children separated from their mothers. Desperation led to unthinkable acts. One day when a deportation list was announced, two women took their babies to an upper floor and threw them out the window, and then flung themselves to their deaths as well. The SS ordered the bodies to be left where they lay, Dr. Odic wrote.

In September 1943, Brunner took Drucker and two other doctors to work in a detention center in Nice, set up in the Hotel Excelsior, treating those whose interrogations had nearly killed them. Brunner commanded a team of a dozen torturers whose goal was to get the names and addresses of family members and associates from their victims. Any and all types of brutality were employed. Drucker and his fellow doctors were ordered to keep the patients alive, in order to extend their suffering. Some of them begged him to help them die.

"During the three months I was detained at the Excelsior, I was witness to and victim of terror and horrible atrocities," Drucker wrote. "Among the arrested were the ill, the infirm, elderly, babies, pregnant women, and all were subject to the violence and torture of these brutes. Most of them were torn from their beds and brought in nightclothes, shivering with fear and cold. Day and night, a large number of the arrested needed medical care, bandages for wounds, for gunshots in the thigh, leg or rear, cut scalps, an ear torn off by the blow of a gun butt, internal bleeding and multiple bruising all over the body, broken teeth, split lips, scraped faces, broken ribs, sprains, etc."[8]

One man was beaten into a coma, with internal bleeding, but when Drucker repeatedly requested to send him to a hospital, Brunner refused. "Not until he talks," Brunner said. He went to the prisoner's room to check on him, saw that the man was unconscious. "He's a faker, he needs to talk," Brunner said.[9] The man died without regaining consciousness. He didn't talk.

The doctors returned to Drancy in December, and they were held there until the German overseers fled and the camp was liberated on August 18, 1944. After the war, Drucker began practicing medicine in Normandy. His elder son Michel became a renowned television star, and his younger son Jacques a public health doctor and epidemiologist. Drucker died in 1983.

While Drancy was the primary transit camp in France, about two hundred other camps also had been set up to hold prisoners of various nationalities. Some were imprisoned on the basis of race, religion, politics, or other perceived offenses of identity, while others were arrested for resistance activity.

From the start of the Occupation in 1940, British civilians caught in France were arrested and sent to an internment camp in Saint Denis, a northern suburb of Paris. Eventually the women were moved to Vittel, a spa town in the east of France. By 1942, an average of three thousand British and some American women were imprisoned in six hotels in Vittel, later joined by Jewish prisoners from Poland and elsewhere in four other hotels. The entire complex of hotels and grounds was surrounded by barbed-wire fences and patrolled by German soldiers. Conditions were far better than in the concentration camps in Germany, with enough food to eat, and health services at a clinic run by two French prisoners-of-war, Dr. Jean Lévy and Dr. René Pigache. After a group of 280 Polish Jews arrived at Vittel in May 1943, camp doctors conspired with a handful of British women prisoners to help them escape. Many of the new arrivals held passports from Latin American nations, but the Germans had refused to recognize them. Among other ruses of resistance, Dr. Lévy was cited by a prisoner as having helped one of the Polish women fake paralysis in order to avoid deportation to Auschwitz.[10]

During the 1940 fighting, the French Army had set up a field hospital in Vittel's Hotel Continental, renamed *Hôpital Complémentaire Continental,* and the Germans took it over as a hospital for prisoners-of-war after the surrender. However most French prisoners-of-war were then transferred to *stalags* in Germany, leaving behind only a Senegalese artillery unit and Martiniquais soldiers—African or African-descended—at Vittel, put to work maintaining the camp.

Racism as the foundation of Nazi beliefs targeted Africans and African Americans as well as Jews, though in different ways. Some Black Americans living in France, many of them stars on the burgeoning jazz scene, were imprisoned from the beginning of the Occupation, when the Nazis outlawed mixed-race or Black performances in cafés and clubs. Among them was Grenada-born trumpetist Arthur Briggs, first sent to Compiègne but transferred to the Saint Denis camp for British prisoners at the request of a fellow musician. They formed an orchestra there that grew to twenty-five members and performed concerts regularly—although jazz and swing were declared "degenerate" music, *verboten.* Banjo and guitar player Maceo Jefferson, who had toured with Louis Armstrong around Europe and married a French woman, drove a truck for the American Hospital of Paris during the Battle for France, moving supplies between Paris and the field hospital at Angoulême. He then went to work for the American Red Cross, and continued composing and recording until December 1941, when the United States entered the war.

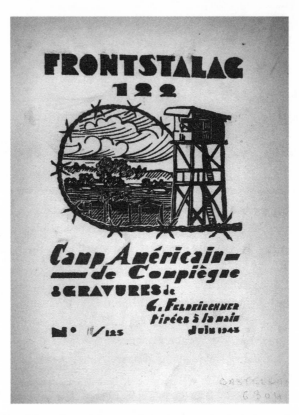

Poster of Compiègne internment camp, drawn by American prisoner
George Feldkirchner. Collection of the Mémorial de l'Internement
et la Déportation, Camp de Royallieu, Compiègne.

At that point, an American section was created in the internment camp
at Compiègne, a former army barracks of twenty-four bunkers called Camp
Royallieu. It contained five other sections—for French political, Russian,
Jewish, women, and high-status prisoners such as former government
officials—overseen by the German Wehrmacht. Within a month of the US
declaration of war, 197 American citizens were interned at Compiègne,
designated by the Germans as Frontstalag 122. Maceo Jefferson and trumpetist Harry Cooper, from Kansas, were among them. They formed a band
with other imprisoned musicians and organized a concert in February 1942.
Cooper managed to get an early release; Jefferson stayed until March 1944.
After the war, he and his wife moved to the United States. He had already
written the song: "Au revoir, pays de mes amours." A group of Latin Ameri-

cans shared the American section, and included a Cuban doctor, Dr. Soler, and a Brazilian dentist, Dr. de Barros.

Prisoners wrote that the different camp sections were by no means equal. The high-status prisoners had the best treatment, the Jews the worst. The American section was considered to be livable, if far from comfortable, with prisoners allowed to receive family visits as well as food packages. The Jewish section, the smallest in the camp, was barred from receiving food packages, and what nutrients the prisoners were provided were doled out at starvation level. An intense black market in food sprang up.

Playwright and author Jean-Jacques Bernard, arrested in December 1941 in a roundup of some seven hundred high-profile Jewish Frenchmen, wrote that he was once offered a tin of sardines for 350 FF (ordinarily sold at fixed price for about 3 FF). He was starving, and at fifty-two years old, starting to collapse when he was given a place in the camp clinic. Each section had a sort of infirmary, but the Russian section held the main clinic, overseen by Dr. Simon Lubicz, a Russian-born immigrant to France who had earned a medical degree in Bordeaux. Lubicz had been imprisoned there since June 1941. Bernard noted that his body temperature hovered around 34°C (93°F), well below normal, and that he could not find the strength to do much more than lie in bed. But the soup in the Russian camp, fare for clinic patients as well, was rich in vegetables, and a precious second serving was on offer, as Bernard discovered upon his arrival. "That night I was almost happy," he wrote. "That infirmary, despite its insufficiencies, seemed to us an oasis. We aspired only to stay there."[11] Bernard recovered slowly through the early winter months of 1942, and he was released from the camp in March. He had lost twenty kilos.

"I will never forget the devotion of Doctor Lubicz," Bernard wrote. "I will never forget the evenings when, before going to sleep, he came to make a last round of the wards, staying sometimes until nearly midnight, listening to the breathing of those who slept, stopping for a minute before those who did not sleep, sitting sometimes on one of our beds, talking for a while in a low voice, bringing to one or another reassurance and comfort. This doctor-prisoner, separated for long months from those he loved, knew how to elevate his thankless task to the level of a mission."[12]

Lubicz seemed to always have the devil on his heels. He had emigrated from Grodno, in what is today Belarus, to escape anti-Jewish pogroms there. In France, he ran up against the strict rules against foreign-born doctors practicing, but when the war broke out, he joined and served in the rugged French Foreign Legion. He was taken prisoner of war with the surrender in June 1940, then held in a German POW camp until April 1941. He was not home two months before the German-Soviet pact ended, and he was arrested as a Russian citizen. After fifteen months at Compiègne, Lubicz was transferred to Drancy and then deported to Auschwitz, where he worked first in a digging detail and then as a body carrier. Sent to the subcamp Buna-Monowitz, set up for slave labor by the IG Farben chemical company, he found work in the infirmary, helping patients avoid selection for the gas chamber. His work there also drew praise from prisoners.

"Not only did he work at treating the exhausted prisoners with the ridiculously meager means at his disposal, but at the risk of his own existence (prisoner-doctors were hanged at Auschwitz for the same reason, to set the example, before all the assembled prisoners), on many occasions he succeeded in removing them from the German 'medical commission' [list] sending them to the gas chamber, prisoners whom he wanted at all costs to see survive in order to testify," wrote one such patient, Zvi Michaéli, a Greek who immigrated to Israel after the war.[13] Michaéli wrote that he had had pneumonia, and Lubicz managed to keep him in the clinic for two weeks, until he was strong enough to work. If he had collapsed, he would have been dispatched to the gas chamber.

With the approach of the Soviet army in January 1945, Auschwitz and its 44 subcamps were emptied and prisoners marched and transported west. Lubicz landed at the Dora subcamp of Buchenwald until April 1945 when, with the Allies closing in, he was among thousands of prisoners sent on death marches northward. Having been an inmate in eight camps over the previous five years, Lubicz survived them all, and finally returned to France in June 1945. He went back to Bordeaux to practice medicine. Zvi Michaéli found him there in 1994. He and some other former camp inmates had a small but joyous reunion. "It's unbelievable," Michaéli wrote. "Fifty years later, I met the doctor who saved me."[14]

The first train to Auschwitz left from Compiègne on March 27, 1942, carrying 1,112 Jewish prisoners, nineteen of whom survived. The last convoy of prisoners left on August 18, 1944, nine days before the camp was liberated, headed for Buchenwald. In between, some fifty thousand men and women—Jews and Resistance fighters and both—were deported from Compiègne to German concentration camps. At Auschwitz alone, more than 1.1

million people died, most of them put to death in the gas chamber.[15] Dr. André Cain, the former chief of gastroenterology at Saint Antoine's Hospital, was among them. After hiding in the south of France since fleeing Paris in fall 1941, Cain and his wife Jeanne were arrested in March 1944. Both were deported to Auschwitz and, according to witnesses, sent directly to the gas chamber. After the war, several colleagues wrote glowing tributes to Cain. His brother Julien Cain, director of the French National Library, survived deportation to Buchenwald.

Four prisoners who did not get deported had Dr. André Marsault, a dermatologist, to thank for it. Arrested in August 1941 for resistance activity (such as possessing a cache of 60 Lebel rifles) near Poitiers, Marsault was sent to Compiègne in April 1942. He worked as a doctor in the clinic, treating his fellow prisoners, until June 17, 1944, when the camp commandant demanded that four of his patients be put on the list for deportation. Marsault refused, insisting that they were too ill to travel. The commandant said fine, then you'll take their place. Marsault was put on the train to Dachau the next day. There, he continued his work as a doctor.[16]

"It was rudely courageous [of him]," wrote Edmond Michelet, a Dachau prisoner who went on to become defense minister of France, in a memoir. "He took care of Block 7, treating erypseles and other skin infections in the company of Dr. Kredit, a Dutch doctor who died of typhus. At one point we feared the worst for Marsault, but tough guys like him don't let themselves be taken down easily."[17]

Marsault survived deportation and returned to his practice in a Paris suburb. Others were not so fortunate: Michelet cited with regret thirteen Dachau prisoner-doctors who died within days of each other after working through a camp epidemic. Michelet had nothing but praise for the French doctors at Dachau. "They treated without medicine, without thermometers, without the least possibility of preventative measures, they wrestled down the epidemics, fighting on every front, determined, tireless—temerity to the point of imprudence."[18]

Another doctor who took a moral stand also found herself deported. Dr. Adélaïde Hautval, a psychiatrist, was arrested in May 1942 trying to cross the demarcation line to visit her ill mother. Sent to jail for a number of weeks as punishment, she watched as hundreds of Jews were imprisoned after mass arrests. When two Gestapo agents came to get a young woman who shared her cell, Hautval spoke out to try to protect her. "'Well, then,

since you defend them, you will share their fates,'" she recounted them saying. "Some days later, they gave me a Jewish star with a sign 'Friend of Jews,'
with orders to sew both of them on my coat."[19] She was transferred to the
French Beaune-la-Rolande internment camp, where she worked as a doctor while imprisoned. Friends and even the Medical Order tried to get her
released, but the price of freedom was not one Hautval was willing to pay:
she refused to rescind her support for the Jewish prisoners. She then was
deported to Auschwitz in January 1943. There, she was asked to treat Block
10 patients, on whom nefarious experiments were conducted. She did so for
four months. But when they asked her to participate in experiments by providing anesthesia for operations to sterilize women, she refused. "I could
not stop myself from saying that no one has the right to dispose of people's
lives in this way," she wrote.[20]

The head doctor at Auschwitz, Eduard Wirths, called her in to his office.
They are Jews, they are different from you, he told her. "In this camp, you
are the one who is different from me," she replied. She expected reprisal, but
instead was transferred back to the women's camp at Birkenau, and eventually to Ravensbrück. In 1965, Hautval testified in a libel trial brought by a
Polish doctor against *Exodus* author Leon Uris, who in his book described
the man as a willing participant in macabre surgical experiments. The doctor's defense was that he had had no choice. Hautval, daughter of an Alsatian
Protestant pastor, told the court that clearly, everyone had a choice. "What
I did was perfectly natural, logical and derived from a moral obligation," she
said later.[21]

"If we had had more friends like Dr. Hautval, there could never have
been a Nazi era," Leon Uris remarked.[22]

7

PRISONERS OF HATRED

Doctors were among nearly 165,000 people arrested in France for Resistance activity and for Jewish or other identity motives and deported to concentration camps in Germany. In the brutality of the camps, their medical skills often saved them from debilitating work details, and they in turn were able to help their fellow prisoners. The doctors' situations evolved over time. At first kept away from medical care, they were eventually allowed to practice with what means they were given or could steal. Among the more than forty thousand prison and internment camps, some were equipped with infirmaries—*Reviers*—of various sizes and personnel, part of the Nazi aim to squeeze as much work as possible out of prisoners before sending them to die.[1] This chapter will focus on the Buchenwald *Konzentrationslager,* where more than eighty French doctors were sent between 1942 and 1944.[2]

Buchenwald—the beech woods—had been set up as a prison camp in 1937 to detain German criminals, communists, and antifascists. With the German annexation of Austria in 1938, the camp's population rose to more than ten thousand prisoners, then nearly doubled with the intensified persecution of Jews across the territory of the Reich. From late 1938, Buchenwald held a mix of prisoners: those detained for political activity; those held for identity bias, such as Jews, Roma, and homosexuals; and those imprisoned as common criminals. A color-coded system of triangles, sewn onto the striped gray pajamas prisoners were given to wear, had green for criminals, red for resistance fighters, yellow for Jews, pink for homosexuals, purple for Jehovah's Witnesses. While some French had been deported to

Buchenwald as early as 1940, they did not arrive there in large numbers before late 1943; by early 1944 they numbered more than seventeen thousand. The first French doctor to arrive was Jean Rousset, a dermatologist and professor at the Medical School in Lyon, deported to Buchenwald in 1942 for resistance activity.

When Rousset got to Buchenwald, he was immediately put to work at the infirmary, an unusual step and one that no doubt saved his life. He joined two Czech doctors who had been imprisoned for seven years already, doing a masterful job of negotiating between SS directives of astounding cruelty, their professional consciences, and the hostility of the other prisoners, who saw them as complicit with the camp administration. "Ardent patriots, they had a ferocious hatred of the Germans that our French comrades were wrong to not discover beneath their apparent submissiveness," Rousset wrote in a postwar memoir.[3]

At the time of Rousset's arrival, Buchenwald was dominated by Russian and Polish prisoners and run by longtime German prisoners, many of whom were communists. They were *kapos,* acting as mid-level administrators of the camp, including the clinics, while overseen by SS officers. The camp was split into two sections, Big Camp and Little Camp, the two separated by electric barbed wire, with separate clinics in each. The Big Camp clinic, by 1945, had nine hundred beds in six housing blocks, and included a dental service, pharmacy, laboratory, operating room and pathology lab. It had begun as one cell block under the first camp commandant, Karl-Otto Koch, who was quoted by the early prisoners as saying: "In my camp, there are no ill people. Here people are well, or they are dead."[4] Koch was transferred to a subcamp in 1941, after his corruption and abuse of prisoners became too much even for the SS, who then carried out his execution in April 1945.

The Little Camp clinic, set up as a facility to quarantine incoming prisoners, had three hundred beds in two housing blocks, and was far more crowded. While a total of 265,980 prisoners came through Buchenwald and its one hundred and thirty subcamps between 1937 and 1945, the average population in autumn 1943 was just over 20,000. It would spike within a year, peaking at 110,000 prisoners (including subcamps) in early 1945. Conditions were so overcrowded and pestilent that winter than an estimated 15,000 prisoners died.[5]

The Big Camp clinic was run by a German prisoner named Ernst Busse, a former Communist Party representative to the Reichstag, who was assisted by Otto Kipp, a German communist journalist. They had been detained at Buchenwald since 1937, and by prisoner accounts, both were intelligent and principled, if hardened by their years of camp life. Prior to the arrival of the Czech and French doctors, the SS had appointed any random prisoner to provide treatment. Thus the "chief surgeon" of the Big Camp clinic was a mason named Helmuth, who had once read an anatomy textbook and honed his scalpel skills on Russian prisoners. The "chief surgeon" of the Little Camp clinic was a shoemaker. Dr. Rousset wrote that one day, when they were trying to get one of the French doctors transferred to work at the Big Camp clinic, Ernst Busse responded: "I'm not asking if he is a doctor, I don't care. Tell me he needs to be named in order to be saved. He will learn the job later."[6]

Rousset noted that at first, real doctors were considered a bother in the clinic. "In truth, we were more tolerated there than wanted. And it required, especially of those of us who stayed until the end, a wealth of patience and a world of diplomacy to put up with the vexations and navigate around the pitfalls of all kinds. We were sustained by the idea that we were useful to our comrades."[7]

As more and more doctors arrived, medical services expanded. Radiologist Joseph Brau was given a Siemens X-ray unit that no one had known how to operate. He was assigned a team of three prisoner assistants, among them Aloïs Grimm, an Austrian Jesuit and scholar who later was hanged for instructing and baptizing an SS soldier. Brau and the team mastered the X-ray machine and began interpreting its results in ways that would help the prisoners, particularly in identifying tubercular lung infections that would prevent a prisoner from being assigned to a tough work detail.

In January 1944, a group of more than 5,500 prisoners arrived, most of whom were French and included doctors Victor Dupont, Léon Elmelik, Jean Lansac, Henri Lignerat, Jacques Poupault, Marcel Renet, Charles Richet, and Charles-Jean Odic. All of them had been involved in Resistance networks. As noted in previous chapters, Victor Dupont was a founder of the Vengeance network, and Charles Richet worked with *Ceux de la Libération*. Upon their arrival, most of them were set to grueling physical labor, breaking rock in a stone quarry or digging pits in frozen ground, in the midst of a bitter winter with neither adequate clothing nor proper tools. But little by little, they found places working either in the camp clinics or in cell blocks designated as infirmaries. Charles Richet, sixty-two years old when Rousset managed to get him named head doctor in the Little Camp clinic, wrote in a memoir that he would not have survived much longer.

"I believed, wrongly, that I had plumbed the depths of human misery through two wars and forty years of hospital life, but I found it there in 'exploring' the quarantine barracks in the first trimester of 1945," Richet wrote. "There, it was a horde of beasts crammed in together."[8] The utter desolation of their circumstances, the emptied shell of human relations, took them all by shock, even those who had gone through Compiègne and Drancy.

"Hatred is stupidly sterile; it repairs nothing, it protects nothing, it does nothing but destroy. We deportees lived for years under the weight of that hate," wrote Dr. Charles-Jean Odic in a postwar memoir. "Love, which had occupied so much room in our actions and our thoughts as a social element, was entirely dead."[9]

Survival became their only goal. And yet, even in the darkest of Malthusian moments, many of the doctor-prisoners found ways to give, and in giving, a way to hold onto their identities. Dr. Louis Girard, an ear-nose-and-throat specialist from Paris, also was sixty-two years old when he was sent to dig a tunnel at the Dora subcamp, or *kommando,* in late 1943. It was known as an extermination kommando, with conditions kept at a degree of harshness few were able to survive. But Girard held on, and in February 1944, an SS guard asked if the doctor could operate on a ten-year-old, possibly the guard's child, it wasn't clear. He did so successfully, and the guards set him up afterward with a makeshift clinic in a storeroom. The prisoners called him "Papa" Girard, and he performed fifty-two mastoidectomies (for ear infection spread to the mastoid region of the skull) while prisoner. He survived to return to France, but died shortly after, in 1947. He had been arrested with his daughter, Anise Girard Postel-Vinay, a Resistance agent who was imprisoned at Ravensbrück and after the war became a key figure in deportee associations.

Saving others, whether fellow prisoners or those held dear by the SS, was proving to be the path to salvation for the doctors themselves. Dr. Pierre Couinaud, a surgeon with his own clinic in Normandy, was deported to Neuengamme camp and put to work cleaning in a factory. Couinaud, fifty-three, was on the edge of collapse after standing in formation for an hours-long roll call one night in September 1944. Just then a passing SS officer asked if any of the prisoners were surgeons. Couinaud stepped forward. They gave him a shower, clean pajamas and a meal, and drove him to a nearby women's camp, where a female factory boss had gotten three fingers mangled in a gear. He suspected the woman was the mistress of one of the guards. Couinaud amputated her fingers with care and skill, and the SS transferred him to work as a doctor in the camp clinic.[10]

Abuse and antagonism from the Nazi guards was expected, but when the big group of French arrived at Buchenwald in January 1944, they were surprised to find hostility coming from another source: their fellow prisoners. The majority Russians and Poles, along with the German antifascists, had anticipated that France, a long-held defender of liberty, would fight and defeat the Nazis, and instead it had collapsed into surrender, occupation, and in many cases, collaboration. By their logic, it was partly France's fault that they were there: the nation had not carried out its given mission. The other prisoners punished the French for this failure by stealing their Red Cross packages and anything else they could.

"[The French] carried the weight of all the mistakes committed in international politics, errors that brought great disappointment to men who expected the French, as was their habit, to run to fight for their freedom," wrote Frédéric-Henri Manhès, a former book editor, military base commander, and key Resistance operative, in a postwar account.[11] Manhès, arrested in March 1943, just after meeting with Charles de Gaulle at his London opposition headquarters, arrived at Buchenwald in January 1944. His work had been by the side of Jean Moulin, pulling disparate groups into a National Council of Resistance, no easy task in the fractious field of French opposition. At Buchenwald Manhès, fifty-four, picked up his previous effort, this time trying to organize the prisoners into a defensive resistance. He wrote that he could see that survival would be impossible if the French did not stick together. It did not help that many of the French Resistance members were intellectuals and professionals, easy pickings in the view of the hardened criminal crowd. But they soon found an advantage.

The earliest political prisoners at Buchenwald, the German communists, had organized into an International Committee of resistance from the start, adding members of other nationalities as they arrived. The new French arrivals, even those who weren't communists, would be a good fit. International Committee leader Ernst Busse, *kapo* of the Big Camp clinic, called doctors Brau, Richet, Elmelik, and nurse Roger Poujol into the X-ray room, with a German professor of French translating, to ask if they would join the group. Dr. Victor Dupont also was interviewed at length by Busse and his committee about his anti-Nazi actions and his political views. As for his medical capacity, the most important question he had to answer was whether he would be able to choose who got treatment and who did not, as there was never enough medicine or material for all the patients. They asked: "If there is only one aspirin, you cannot cut it in two, to whom do you give it?"[12]

While on one level the French began organizing to defend themselves as a national group, their involvement with the established and larger committee was key to improving their situation. The International Committee emphasized to the new recruits that the goal was survival: simply by staying alive, they defeated the Nazi program of extermination. Everything they did was aimed at survival. In time, Dupont got Manhès off an arduous digging detail and into the Little Camp clinic, and he was quickly brought into the International Committee as well. Then in May 1944, Marcel Paul, a well-known and respected communist union organizer, arrived at Buchenwald and intensified the French effort, while working closely with the International Committee. Paul and Manhès expanded the French group from about thirty to more than a hundred members, named it the Committee of French Interests, and set two goals: to permit a maximum of French to survive in good condition, and to slow and sabotage the German war production. To that end they managed to move more and more French workers into the weapons and electronics factories at Buchenwald, providing increased opportunity for sabotage. It was dangerous. When a worker was caught leaving the fuses off grenades he was making, committee members had to quickly switch his identity papers with a dead prisoner to save his life.

For the first goal, to survive in good condition, the camp clinics played a major role. Dr. Brau was named to preside over the medical section of the clandestine committee, and he used his special access to food and supplies to help ill prisoners. Before Brau arrived at the Big Camp clinic, only an SS officer could decide whether or not a patient would be admitted—a life-or-death call that the SS based solely on whether or not the prisoner had a fever. Brau managed to take over admissions, conducting an interview and diagnosis before deciding whether to let a prisoner stay.[13] Like the camp, the clinics were vastly overcrowded from 1944 onward, with two to four patients per sixty-centimeter bunk, and others lying in straw on the stone floor. Only one out of every twenty patients who needed hospitalization was admitted. To alleviate conditions, the prisoners' committees persuaded the camp administration to allow a doctor per cell block, so that patients who needed help could receive it in their block as well. And rather than crowd all the diseases and conditions into the same ward, they designated one block for tuberculosis, one for dysentery, another for typhus. Dr. Dupont took over the tuberculosis ward, which was particularly suited for hiding prisoners in trouble, as the German guards were fearful of contagion.

After the war, Dupont wrote a brilliant essay in which he tried to answer the essential question of why, if the Nazis aimed to kill all the prisoners, did they bother to provide care at all? He noted that the intention of the concentration camp system was indeed death for all, but said the Germans could not, in the interest of efficiency, let free labor go to waste. The Gestapo judge who sent him to Buchenwald told him: "It is much more interesting for us to send you to work in Germany than to shoot you."[14]

By January 1944, large factories had been set up to manufacture munitions and rockets conveniently next to the thousands of slave labor camps. While German men were sent to fight in and occupy other nations, the prisoners became the Reich's work force. "They represented exploitable energy that the German spirit could not bear to see lost, especially during a war that called for an enormous effort, unhealthy work (such as digging in the deep galleries of mines, created for underground factories), and, absolutely secret! A completely isolated work force, guarded by personnel fanatically devoted to their masters, offered a maximum guarantee against Allied espionage," Dupont wrote.[15]

Deniability was key to the scheme. The Germans adhered to a script that their justice system was indulgent in allowing enemies to work for them, rather than being executed. After the Allied landing in June 1944, the SS administration began to allow more and more prisoners to take over running the camps, also part of the deniability element, according to Dupont. The International Committee gathered evidence wherever it could to attest to German acts and intentions. It wasn't that difficult to do, as the SS had grown accustomed to casual cruelty and believed their cause of "Aryan" supremacy justified any means.

"This utilitarianism, as a general rule, was aggravated by sadism exhibited in a pure state, through a variety of tortures, but that also justified itself in other domains through pseudo-scientific pretexts," Dupont wrote, adding that the polarized political climate of the time had paved the way for such beliefs. "There was favorable ground for the culture of fanaticism that Hitler and his henchmen knew how to use."[16]

On a medical level, this fanaticism also took the form of using prisoners for torturous medical experiments. The camp medical commander, Gerhard Schiedlausky, had begun sadistic surgical experiments on women prisoners at Ravensbrück camp before being transferred in October 1943 to Buchenwald, where he continued his macabre work. In his testimony at the Nuremberg Trials in 1946, Dr. Dupont said that Schiedlausky had set up a room in the Little Camp clinic in which lethal injections were given to prisoners he wanted out of the way, and another cell block was used to exterminate those who could no longer work. Buchenwald did not have a gas chamber, but bodies "were transported to the crematorium in carts, especially during the roll calls or during the night," Dupont said. In winter of 1945, when the camp's population was at a peak, the Little Camp counted 150 deaths a day. Dupont also was assigned to select prisoners with little or no hope of recovery for extermination by lethal injection. "That order, I never carried out," he testified.[17]

One of the experiments the SS imposed on prisoners at Buchenwald tested vaccines or possible "cures" for typhus, a deadly bacterial disease transmitted by lice. A German doctor, Erwin Ding-Schuler, conducted those, infecting prisoners, testing either a vaccine or various potential "cures," and then executing the prisoners with lethal injections when the "cure" failed. Ding-Schuler committed suicide while in US custody in 1945. Schiedlausky, who made daily rounds of the Big Camp clinic and oversaw its operations closely, was executed in 1947 after being found guilty of war crimes. The camp commander after 1942, Hermann Pister, was charged with war crimes after the war and sentenced to death, but died of a heart attack while still in prison.

After returning home, Charles Richet wrote a memoir that analyzed the social strata in the camp and how conditions differed widely between the groups. At Buchenwald, Richet said the SS left the running of the camp in the hands of about two hundred senior prisoners, such as Ernst Busse. Some of these *kapos* were brutal thugs and some were not, but they had privileges and freedom of movement the other prisoners lacked. Under them, Richet counted about 2,500 prisoners who worked in relative comfort and security, including clinic doctors and nurses. Another 15,000 prisoners slept two to a bed and ate regularly, and some even had shoes. But, he wrote, the great mass of prisoners, as many as 30,000 at times, were stuck in a slow grind toward death, worked to the bone, starving and diseased, nothing in their lives but fear, cold, hunger, and hatred. He noted that 75 percent of his transport convoy, arriving in January 1944, had died in the first eight months.[18]

Like Manhès with political organizing, Richet continued in the camp with work he had been doing outside, observing the effects on the population of nutrition at famine and starvation levels. He calculated that from January 1944 to January 1945, the prisoners were getting about 60 percent of needed calories; ten to twelve hours of physical work per day in the freezing cold required three thousand calories a day. On a daily basis, prisoners were fed a greasy rutabaga soup, five hundred grams of bread or potatoes, a dab of margarine or jam. Once a week they got either 250 grams of skim milk or fish or carrots or beets. No fruit, no green vegetables, thus no iron or calcium. But from January 1945 to liberation, as the Germans' war footing slipped further and further, prisoners' rations were cut in half. By April 1945, they were getting perhaps a thousand calories a day.[19]

Richet also noted the physical consequences of starvation, such as swelling or edema of body parts, and pellagra, which attacked the skin, intestines, and brain due to severe lack of niacin. Disease brought on by overcrowding and insufficiency included pneumonia—he estimated 12 percent of the camp had it at any moment—and dysentery, which a fifth of the prisoners had and which killed 60 percent of its victims. At Ravensbrück, imprisoned doctor Paulette Don Zimmet-Gazel also noted the physical effects of camp conditions, and she wrote a doctoral dissertation on it upon her return.

Richet's report was scientific, observational, astute, and devoid of emotion. Yet, as chief doctor of the Little Camp clinic, he had his share of difficulties. He recounted one incident in April 1944 when four Russian prisoners were sentenced to death, and one of them managed to hide in Richet's clinic. The camp *kapos* ordered him to kill the man. Instead, he charted a fake temperature spike and death, along with a cremation certificate, and sneaked the man out of camp.[20] After the war, Richet devoted himself to researching the pathology of deportation, trying to assess the physical effects of the years of deprivation that prisoners had endured. He personally received a 100 percent disability pension due to injuries and damage sustained in the camps.

Perhaps the most significant day at Buchenwald, before that of liberation, was August 24, 1944, when the US Army Air Corps' 613th Squadron bombed the camp. Its targets were the Gustloff weapons factory, where some twelve thousand workers made G43 rifles; the DAW electronics factory, which made parts for the V2 rockets raining down on London; and the SS barracks. When the air-raid siren wailed shortly before noon, prisoners working in the factories were pleased: it was a regular occurrence, and it meant taking a break. They went to a small wood next to the factory and sat down, ringed by SS guards. But unlike previous flights, the first airplane did not continue in an easterly direction. Instead it circled once and then, with a puff of white smoke, began dropping bombs. The thunderous impact sent shrapnel flying into the woods, and some prisoners tried to flee. Pierre Bretonneau, a French prisoner, wrote that as he and a Russian prisoner jumped up to run, an SS guard shot and killed the Russian; Bretonneau sank back to the ground. With clouds of smoke and dust billowing from the destroyed factories and SS barracks, the planes then scattered a shower of small phosphorus bombs across the forest, setting it aflame. Bretonneau wrote that he was dazed by the screams of burning men and coils of black smoke, when he felt a sharp pain in his leg. He had been hit, his leg shredded and his foot nearly blown off. A fellow prisoner offered his belt as a tourniquet to stop the bleeding, and some other prisoners lifted him onto a stretcher cobbled together from pine branches and carried him to the Big Camp clinic. The wounded lay on the ground to await care; for Bretonneau, the wait was ten hours. The SS doctor then summarily ordered him sent to a room Bretonneau knew to be the antechamber of the crematorium. He was taken there and left to die. Fever and gangrene were rising when at 3 a.m. prisoner stretcher-bearers got him and took him into the clinic. Dr. Pierre Maynadier amputated his leg just below the knee and saved his life.[21] Maynadier and Drs. Paul-Louis Fresnel, Léon Elmelik, and Paul Denis, among others, worked nonstop in relays over the following ten days, treating and operating and doing what they could for the injured, despite a near-total lack of material. Maynadier later reported that he had operated on two thousand patients—prisoners and SS alike—in the week after the bombing. The Germans reported 315 prisoners and 80 SS killed, and some 1,500 guards and prisoners wounded, but most believe the casualty figures were much higher.

The result of the doctors' indefatigable effort, and of the prisoners' having organized a stretcher-bearing service in the heat of the emergency, improved French standing in the camp. In the immediate aftermath of the bombing, there was no electricity, no water, no soup—but nor were there work details and interminable roll calls. Earlier in the summer, the clandestine camp committees had begun to form a military branch, and they took advantage of the postbombing chaos to solidify its structure. The French branch, led by Frédéric-Henri Manhès, called itself the French Brigade of Liberation Action and gained some 2,500 members over the following year. Throughout the camp, members from eleven nations formed three battalions, divided into companies and sections. There were also three commando squadrons. The committees managed to rearrange prisoners from cell block to cell block to consolidate the military units. And the clandestine army was now armed: after the bombing, they had stolen as many guns and weapons as they could from dead guards and hidden them away.[22]

The leaders agreed, after long and considered discussion, that they should take no action that could lead to massacre or reprisal by the SS, unless the situation became critical. The coolest, most rational heads prevailed, at a time when the temptation to act must have been dauntingly strong. They had managed to build a radio receiver from parts stolen from the electronics factory and were able to follow the progress of the fighting. They knew that Paris had been liberated the day after their bombing, and that the Allied forces were continuing eastward. They had the Germans on the run; it was a question of time. But as conditions deteriorated, food became scarcer, and the death toll rose, particularly in the winter of 1945, how did they continue to wait? The numbers remained terrifically against them. Clandestine committees made up a small fraction of the overall camp population, most of whom had no idea of the groups' existence. With the complicity of some of the kapos, the committee members kept their focus on the goal of survival.[23]

In January 1945, several thousand prisoners were evacuated from the Auschwitz camp as the Russian Army approached. They spent eight days in open horse-drawn carts to get to Buchenwald. "There were hundreds dead upon their arrival and the number of deaths in the following days was horrifying," said Dr. Marcel Renet, in a postwar interview. "Many of the prisoners had their feet completely frozen, but were denied access to the hospital and to amputation that would have saved them."[24]

Renet, who had been arrested for resistance work, left medicine after the war and became a journalist and senator. At Buchenwald, he worked for a time in the tuberculosis clinic. "There was not the least medication and the ill received absolutely no treatment," he said. "The mortality rate was about 60 percent per month."

The death toll at Buchenwald spiked from January through March 1945:

2,000 dead in January; 5,400 in February, 5,600 in March. By February, the SS had no more fuel to operate its crematorium ovens, which had been specially designed to incinerate several bodies at once. The bodies stacked up, and the rat population increased, until in March, administrators agreed to bury the dead prisoners in mass graves. Hope, in the midst of cold despair, came in the form of radio reports that American troops were moving eastward across Germany.

The clandestine International Committee met on April 4, and the French urged a camp-wide uprising. The German prisoners refused, insisting that the SS would turn the camp over to the Americans as it was, no need to risk more lives, according to Manhès. Two days later, the SS began forming ranks of prisoners to evacuate the camp, marching into the distance until death. The French put everyone they could into cell block 31, and refused to leave. The SS came on April 10 to kick them out. The French dragged their feet, delaying as much as possible. They went outside to line up, and saw an American plane fly over the camp at low altitude and shoot at the guard tower. The prisoners returned to their cell block; the SS guards began to leave. The officers had already packed up their cars and fled.[25]

The following morning, April 11, the prisoners could hear gunfire. At noon the committee ordered the French prisoner commandos into action, sending them to a cell block where weapons were stashed. On the way they passed a couple of German prisoners next to a pile of coal shoveled against the wall of the SS hospital. They watched as the Germans lit a fuse and bombed open the wall. Inside was an armory of guns and ammunition. The French were given twenty-eight rifles, one machine gun, and two cases of grenades. They were sent to the western side of the camp, where some remaining SS troops had been set up to defend against the Americans' approach. The prisoner commando took out the troops, including some hidden machine-gun nests that could have cost many lives. They then continued through the forest toward the nearby town of Weimar, ready to capture it as well. Instead, they encountered members of the US Third Army's 6th Armored Division, the soldiers wondering at the armed men in striped pajamas. They explained, shook hands, the soldiers handed out cigarettes, and they returned to the camp.

As the larger population of prisoners understood that liberation was finally at hand, they erupted in joy. The German prisoners, some of whom had been there as long as eight years, simply wept. It was over, and they had survived. Frédéric-Henri Manhès wrote in his account: "We had just one word to say: *Merci.*"[26]

The following day, members of the US 80th Infantry Division arrived to take control of the camp. Dr. Brau was named camp doctor and given supplies to treat the desperately ill. Journalists were brought in to record the horrifying conditions of the camp, and General George S. Patton, commander of the US Third Army, ordered the citizens of Weimar to walk to the camp and take a good hard look at what had been going on under their noses. Dr. Michel Léon-Kindberg, sixty-one, who had survived the transfer from Auschwitz in January, said in a report that Weimar had sent a team of flame-throwers with orders to destroy the camp and kill anyone left in it. They were stopped in the nick of time by the arrival of the American troops. "If the Americans had arrived an hour and a half later, the whole camp would have been burned, and they would have found only charred bones," he said.[27]

A week later, Drs. Richet, Elmelik, and Léon-Kindberg, along with Manhès and Marcel Paul, were among forty-three former prisoners on the first transport back to Paris, landing at Le Bourget Airport on April 18. Dr. Toussaint Gallet, a gynecologist who had spent nine months at Buchenwald, also was on the plane. He took the next day off to see his family, and then on April 20 he began working as medical supervisor at the Lutetia Hotel. The historic hotel, seized as Abwehr headquarters during the Occupation, now served as the city's reception center for deportees, in all imaginable conditions, flooding back from the camps to France. At Gallet's funeral in 1970, a fellow doctor and former prisoner spoke of his time at Buchenwald:

"A doctor he remained in the jungle of the camp, a doctor with bare hands who could not treat the body, but a doctor to the lost, the weak, and to those who had given up," said Dr. Henri Parlanges. "How many of us found, thanks to him, the hope or simply the indispensable calm to continue to 'hold on'? How many felt stronger for having shared his strength, soothed because he could communicate his serenity? Help in overcoming weakness often meant saving a life. Many of us returned only because we had the luck, at a decisive moment, to meet an exceptional human being like our friend Gallet."[28]

Much the same was said of the other doctors who worked at Buchenwald to keep their fellow prisoners alive. Gallet became president of the Association of Deported Doctors after the war, a group that counted several hundred former prisoners and internees. Most of them went back to their medical careers, and some also became active in local and national politics.

For other former prisoners, postwar life did not turn out so well. Ernst Busse, the communist International Committee leader, became interior minister of Thuringia province, part of Soviet-occupied Germany. Then, accused by former Russian prisoners of not having done enough for them at Buchenwald, he resigned. In 1950, he was invited to a meeting in Berlin with a Soviet official, arrested on the spot, and sent to Moscow. After surviving eight years at Buchenwald, it was his fate to die in a gulag, in 1952.

8

BLOOD IN THE FOREST

Some doctors who were deeply involved in resistance work avoided arrest and deportation by escaping to join rural guerrillas known as *maquisards,* from the Corsican term for those in trouble who took to the bush rather than surrender to the authorities. All across France from 1942 on, increasing numbers of young people were setting up secret guerrilla camps to avoid being sent to Germany to work, and to prepare for the battle to end the Nazi Occupation. This chapter will examine the Morvan Forest maquisards and their medical team.

On May 30, 1944, Dr. Alec Prochiantz took a bus 270 kilometers (168 miles) south from Paris to the town of Nevers, carrying a suitcase full of medical supplies and 5,000 FF in cash given to him by Dr. Paul Milliez on behalf of the Committee of Medical Resistance (CMR). His contact in Nevers was a pharmacist, who then joined him on a short bus ride east to the village of Ouroux-en-Morvan, in the heart of the Morvan Forest. The Morvan, five thousand square kilometers (1,930 square miles) of old oak, birch, chestnut, and elm trees, had neither highways nor train tracks traversing it. The terrain was hilly but not mountainous, rather a plateau with scattered farms and villages but no large towns. It was the perfect place to hide burgeoning encampments of guerrilla fighters.

The CMR sent Prochiantz, a thirty-year-old medical resident from Paris, to provide care for the Morvan maquisards, whose assigned task was to tie up Nazi forces in the center of France in preparation for D-Day. First, he had to get there. A German member of the *Feldgendarmerie* stopped the bus he was on and inspected the papers of its passengers and the bags they carried. During his inspection, the officer sat on a suitcase, the one bag he

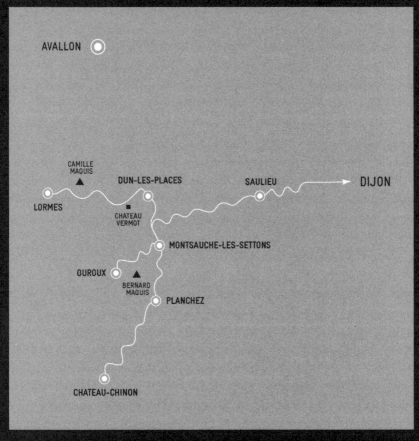

Map of the Morvan plateau showing maquisard camps and towns.
Anastasia Komnou.

neglected to look into. It was Prochiantz's, and had he opened it, Prochiantz would have been taken on the spot. As it was, three other passengers were taken off the bus and arrested. At Ouroux, a driver picked him up and drove him into the forest to the guerrilla camp. Prochiantz's fiancée, Edmée Rodrigues, joined him the following week via the same route. They had met in medical school, and she now was specializing in anesthesiology. In the bush, everyone went by code names, and theirs were Monsieur de Martell and Madame de Martell. Prochiantz wrote nonchalantly that it was after the brand of cognac, that Courvoisier had already been taken.[1]

First, they stayed in a house in a village not far from Montsauche-les-Settons, but the traffic of people coming and going for treatment became too obvious. They left just in time, watching from a hidden distance as German police sacked the house, looking for them. Into the forest they fled, staying in the camp of the "Camille" group. Each camp had its own name, often that of the pseudonym of the leader. By June 1944, the Morvan hosted three to five thousand maquisards, divided into a dozen groups. They had started small—the Camille group had five men in 1942—and had grown as Vichy's Obligatory Work Service (STO) intensified, requiring forced labor in Germany of most young men in France. Instead, the targeted men slipped into hiding on isolated farms, in mountain areas, or in forests like the Morvan. As they became organized bands of guerrillas, they developed contacts with the Free French organization in London, which supplied them with weapons, clothes, medical supplies, canned food, cash, and even vehicles, parachuted in drops beginning in November 1942. By the time Prochiantz arrived, the Morvan guerrillas had extensive camps, landing areas for airplanes, a fleet of vehicles, and an armory that ranged from rusty pistols to modern artillery.

But they didn't have a hospital. Local doctors, including Dr. Léon Bondoux, who also was mayor of Chateau-Chinon, one of the Morvan's larger villages (with 2,400 residents), helped the guerrillas as best they could, but there were German police watching them. If injured men came to town for treatment, they risked arrest, or worse. After the June 6th Allied landing in Normandy, the Morvan guerrillas launched Operation *Hérisson* (Hedgehog), aimed at delaying Germans' transport in central France to prevent them from reinforcing troops in Normandy. They were to carry out sabotage missions on train tracks, roads, and bridges, and to launch ambushes on German troops. There would be wounded to treat.

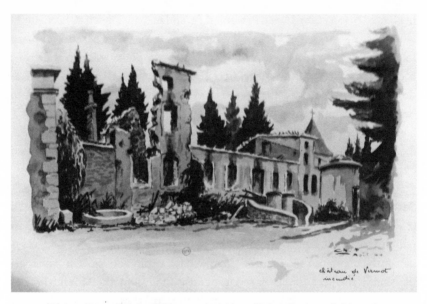

Watercolor painting of the maquisard hospital at Chateau de Vermot
in the Morvan, by Sgt. Blémus, whose *nom de guerre* was "Cherbourg."
Bibliothèque Nationale de France.

The Camille group of guerrillas showed Prochiantz an empty manor house where he could set up a clinic. The Chateau de Vermot sat on a small departmental road outside the village of Dun-les-Places. Spacious, occupied only by a caretaker, it was rapidly furnished with beds, an operating table with lamps rigged from car headlights, a pressure-cooker for rapid sterilization of instruments, and parts to rig up a traction device. The National Resistance representative, André Rondenay (pseudonym Jarry), had even brought an X-ray machine from a nearby hospital, but as no one knew how to run it, it wasn't used. Prochiantz wrote that it was practically like working in a hospital. Their first patient was a guerrilla accidentally shot by a jumpy guard when he returned to camp.

A male nurse from the hospital at Nevers drove Prochiantz around in a Renault Viva Grand Sport, an elegant model the nurse had "requisitioned" from a Vichy government motor pool and decorated with a large double-barred cross of Lorraine, symbol of the Free French. Packed with emergency medical instruments and material, and fueled by wood alcohol (methanol), the medical service car traveled from camp to camp to treat injured men around the Morvan, taking the back roads to avoid German patrols.

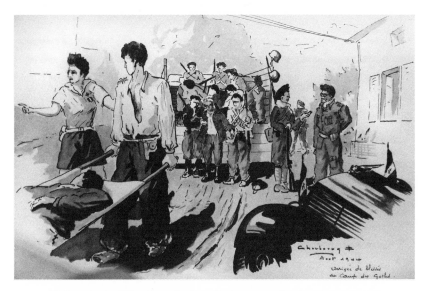

Watercolor by "Cherbourg" of medical personnel caring for wounded
maquisards in the Morvan. Bibliothèque Nationale de France.

Health troubles stemmed not only from armed conflict: conditions were
rough, infections set in, the damp chill of the forest—that summer's weather
was described by British officers as somewhere between "appalling" and
"atrocious"[2]—led to bronchitis, and the lack of bathing facilities brought on
an outbreak of scabies in one camp. While they usually had enough food, it
was not particularly nutritious. The maquisards bought food from the local
farms, or ate canned K-rations. Their diet was meat, potatoes, eggs, cheese.
No vegetables or fruit. And Prochiantz himself complained to leaders of one
camp about its set-up: "The kitchen is about ten meters from the slaugh-
terhouse. The livestock, once slaughtered, the carcasses are barely buried."
Maggots accompanied a permanent odor of decay, and the washing-up station right next to the well meant the men were bathing in water also used for
drinking and cooking, Prochiantz wrote.[3]

That description of filth and disorder is also an indication of the number of women in the camps: not many. Edmée Rodrigues and a female student nurse worked with Prochiantz, and some of the other camps counted
a couple of nurses, a woman doctor, or a few nuns who had volunteered to
join the maquisards. In the Camille group, the sister of one of the founders,
Françoise Longhi (pseudonym Lucette), ran the infirmary, assisted by her

thirteen-year-old daughter, Giselle. They moved to the Chateau de Vermot when the clinic was set up there. Historians estimate that only about 10 percent of the maquisards were women, less than in other Resistance organizations. However the key role of liaison between camps was carried out almost exclusively by local women, riding bicycles on back-country roads to carry messages from one group to another, using food supply and other errands as cover for their trips.

In early June 1944, a British SAS (Special Air Services, formed in 1941) team that would eventually number sixty men began parachuting into the area. One SAS paratrooper, Bill Burgess, fractured his leg severely upon landing on June 22. On the same landing, another SAS paratrooper wrenched his back and could not walk.[4] Burgess and Sgt. Frederick "Chalky" White were driven to Chateau de Vermot, where Prochiantz diagnosed Sgt. White, without benefit of an X-ray, with broken lower-back vertebrae. On June 26, the nurse-driver and Prochiantz left to take Burgess for a discreet X-ray at the hospital in Saulieu, twenty-two kilometers east, where doctors had helped them on emergency cases before. Sgt. White was lying in bed at Chateau de Vermot about 6 p.m. when suddenly a burst of machine-gun fire riddled the wall above his head. The Germans were attacking the hospital. White jumped up and ran, along with the other patients, a doctor and nurses, some carrying patients on stretchers, one hundred meters to the tree line of the forest. (Prochiantz wrote later, wryly, that along with the hospital, he lost all confidence in his diagnostic acumen.[5] Patients with broken back vertebrae do not run, no matter how frightened.) What had blown the secrecy of the clandestine clinic?

Earlier that day, the Bernard group of guerrillas had ambushed a German convoy on the road to Vermot, using explosive mines to demolish a couple of trucks and shooting at the rest of the vehicles from positions on a hill above the road. The Germans, with a force of about 250 troops, then attacked the clinic, launching fire bombs to set it aflame. An urgently sent message brought the help of an SAS squadron, which closed in on the Germans as they filed back up the road, killing forty to fifty of them. One SAS man was shot in the neck, but survived. Meanwhile, seeing unanticipated German troop movements around him as he drove, Prochiantz decided it was too risky to try to get Burgess into Saulieu and had turned around to return to Vermot. He saw the flames of the burning clinic from a high point on the road.

After destroying the clinic, the German troops advanced to the village of Vermot and burned it to the ground, shooting six inhabitants dead. Then, about 7:30 p.m., a contingent of some 400 Germans pulled into the main square at Dun-les-Places, a nearby village of about eight hundred residents. These Germans were not simple soldiers. The group, which grew to number nearly three thousand, included commanders in the regional SD (*Sicherheitsdienst*) police, the intelligence branch that seconded the Gestapo, from garrisons in Dijon and Chalon-sur-Sâone; Wehrmacht Army soldiers of the Ost Battalion 654, many of whom were of Russian origin; and some French militia thugs. Soldiers rousted the men of the village—the mayor, the schoolteacher, and the priest among them—and held them at gunpoint in the town center, in front of the church. Troops surrounded the town with armored trucks and set up artillery guns at the crossroads. The interrogation began: Where were the maquisards hiding? Where was the SAS camp? No one responded. The priest was ordered to climb the bell tower.[6]

"The enemy claimed to have been fired on by civilians from the church tower. This was demonstrably untrue, as every civilian who was armed was with the Maquis, and there were no Maquisards in Dun that day," wrote one of the SAS troopers, Ian Wellsted.[7]

The killing began. Soldiers bludgeoned the priest to death, leaving his body on the stairs to the bell tower. Then they opened fire with automatic rifles and threw grenades into the group, killing twenty-six of the men. Women and children of the town had been told to stay in their houses, some in their cellars. They heard the gunfire and feared the worst. At the same time, a fierce storm erupted in crashing bouts of lightning and thunder, and the electric power went out.

"But through the growling of the storm, we heard the bursts of automatic weapons. Shouts pierced the fracas, cries: the men howled. I never knew what it was they cried," René Marin wrote in a memoir seventy years later. He had been a seven-year-old boy, sent with his mother to a cellar across the street from the massacre. His father was among those shot. "Even today, the thought of it sends chills down my spine. I have forgotten nothing."[8]

The troops spent the rest of the night drinking, dancing in the streets to an accordion, and pillaging the village, before burning to the ground a dozen homes. Then they moved on to Montsauche-les-Settons, a village of about a thousand residents ten kilometers south, and burned it as well. As they left, they were ambushed by a group of maquisards, who managed to kill seventeen Germans. But the bulk of the troops continued on to the village of Planchez, another ten kilometers south, and torched it. In Montsauche and Planchez, several local men were shot and killed. The first of the Bernard guerrillas also was killed in the fighting. Jacques "Jacky" Chataigneau, a twenty-four-year-old student, was shot in the first ambush. Prochiantz had known him in Paris; he was part of the Vengeance network. In the Morvan, he had worn an old Scout uniform. His death hit them all hard, bringing into focus the very real risks they ran. "We just didn't realize," Prochiantz said in an interview years later. "We were turned toward life, not death."[9]

The attacks were part of the German response to the Allied landings in Normandy. While battles raged between armies to the north, German soldiers—often accompanied by French militiamen—assaulted small, defenseless towns and villages in the rest of the country. French civilians had been targets throughout the Occupation, but the summer of 1944 was a particularly murderous time. In central France, on June 10 in the town of Oradour-sur-Glane, German troops of the 2nd Panzer division locked more than 600 residents, including 247 children, inside a church and set it on fire. All of them died. In the eastern Alps, a large group of maquisards had asked their team of doctors to hide more than 120 wounded in the forest, as a German sweep was on its way. The medical group took refuge in La Luire cave on the Vercors plateau on July 21. Some of the doctors and patients moved on the next day, but three doctors, nine nurses, and a Jesuit priest stayed with nearly thirty patients who could not walk. The Germans arrived, shot fourteen of them, put another dozen in a truck, and sent it to Grenoble. Two of the doctors—both Jews who had been forced out of their Paris practices— were executed there, though a third managed to escape. The nurses were arrested and deported to Ravensbrück concentration camp. One of the nurses, Anita Winter, was asked in 1954 by the Vercors maquisard commander to recount what had happened that day. She wrote that the Germans had split them into groups and sent one group ahead. When the second group heard the burst of machine-gun fire, the men knew what awaited them. "They stood straight and proud and shouted to me: 'Tell our families, tell my wife, tell my children that we carried on to the end, we did what we could, you'll tell them, you'll tell them . . .' I can still hear them and I weep in writing these lines."[10]

The Morvan was in the path of the Germans' eastward movement, and its small groups of guerrillas and teams of SAS were not enough to put a stop to the marauding and massacre. After the attack on Dun-les-Places,

Prochiantz spent three days trying to find the SAS encampment in the forest near Vermot. He begged the commander to take on the defense of the Montsauche SAS team, being hunted by the Germans, but the commander asked him to count the troops at his disposal: forty men. All he could do for the moment was hide, and wait.[11] Prochiantz meanwhile had wounded to treat, and nowhere to do so, now that Chateau de Vermot was gone. When a young maquisard was accidentally shot in the stomach at close range, there was nothing to do but drive him to the hospital at Saulieu and hope for help. They found it: the supervising nun showed them to the operating room, and the chief surgeon came to assist. They posted guards outside the door. The young man died on the table, his intestines had been shattered, and the hospital had no material for resuscitation, not even physiological serum. They took his body back to the camp for burial.

The maquisards, in the meantime, began receiving the latest in modern pharmaceuticals in their parachute drops. Morphine in syringes, brand-new Pentothal for anesthesia, even penicillin, whose industrial production had just begun in the United States. They had the equipment, but they had to improvise the clinics. Operations often took place on a farmer's kitchen table. Prochiantz recounted having operated more than once at the Renault farm, on the edge of the forest a few kilometers south of Montsauche. "Afterward, the patients installed in Renault family beds, the smell of cooking, for our pleasure, would replace the odor of chloroform," he wrote.[12] But repeated use put the Renault family in danger, and Prochiantz wanted a safer solution.

The Bernard camp provided it. Led by Louis Aubin, a retired gendarme and municipal councillor at Montsauche, the Bernard group held the most central camp in the Morvan. It was the second iteration of the Bernard group, now counting a hundred men, after the first one was dissolved in the face of fierce German reprisal. Working with the mayor's office at Montsauche, Louis Aubin had sabotaged a German-ordered livestock roundup in October 1943 and had returned the animals to their owners. In so doing, he had reaped a harvest of gratitude from the local farmers. Then in November 1943, Aubin led a parade on Armistice Day to the town's monument to its Great War dead, laying a flower wreath in the form of a Lorraine cross. These two daring acts of public resistance brought down German fury, and he and the others had to go into hiding "with the sympathy of the peasants and the respect of the patriots."[13] Another Armistice Day parade that year, in the eastern Jura mountain town of Oyonnax, saw some 200 maquisards march through and place a Lorraine-cross wreath at the town monument, with a message to past and future: "From the victorious of tomorrow to those of 14–18." One of the guerrillas filmed the march, the surprised townspeople applauding and cheering them on; they sent the film to London, where Free French officials shared it with the Allies.[14] It was solid evidence that on the ground, people were ready to fight back.

By early summer of 1944, the Allies were dropping equipment by the ton by parachutes. Historian Jacques Canaud noted the irony in the fact that the most modern of transport methods, the airplane, was being used to get equipment to men who then had to resort to the most ancient of transport methods, the ox cart, to move them.[15] When the guerrillas received radio notice that a drop was scheduled, they set up car headlights attached to batteries in a triangle to outline the drop zone, often a potato field. Men waited to signal to the planes with flashlights. SAS trooper Ian Wellsted wrote in his memoir about the symphony of a night drop: "As it passed the first light there came a swish and crack of opening chutes, and a clang-clang as the containers bumped together."[16] The containers, stuffed with everything from canned beans to sabotage explosives, medicine to fishing poles, cash to toilet paper, weighed as much as 250 kilos (550 pounds) each. The men needed teams of oxen to get the material back to the camps.

"How we relied upon these sturdy hard-working folk and their heavy oxen, who used to pull overloaded wooden carts up the deeply rutted tracks into the heart of our woods. None of them ever betrayed us," Wellsted wrote.[17]

Loyalty was no doubt strong, but the money sent by the Allies also was insurance against betrayal. The guerrillas were getting about 70 million francs ($243,000 at the black market rate) a month, dropped in million-franc packages to the Camille group, which was responsible for distributing it to the other groups in the Morvan.[18] The cash was used to buy supplies from the local farmers, to pay for fuel and services by local mechanics, and by the summer of 1944, to give the men some minimal wages (10 FF per day), most of which went to helping support their families while they were in hiding.

The supply drops rarely were smooth. Of the Jeeps parachuted to the maquis, several crashed ("pranged" in SAS parlance) and could not be used. On July 5, two Jeeps landed well but a third came down in a wooded grove, and forty trees had to be cut down to get it out. Wellsted wrote that when there was a drop, at least thirty men would spend the entire night finding the scattered containers and dragging them to a consolidated spot under a tree.[19] At daylight farmers with ox carts would arrive to load up and transport the material, hiding it under stacks of hay.

Nonetheless the drops of hundreds of containers sometimes drew the attention of the Germans. A week before the July massacres on Vercors plateau, seventy-two Allied planes had dropped more than a thousand containers. On July 14, thirty-five planes dropped nine hundred containers to maquisards in the Haute Vienne department, and three days later, the Germans attacked them there.[20] On July 18, in the northern sector of the Morvan, an American and a British plane collided when both attempted to make a drop in the same zone. All sixteen crew members were killed. The next day, German police asked the mayor of Mazignen village what the loud noise had been. The guerrillas told him to say one plane had crashed.

All of those drops were by parachute, and as nothing went to waste in those hard years, their silk, cotton, or nylon material was re-used in a variety of ways, cut up for handkerchiefs, scarves, bandages, even altar cloths. The maquisards particularly appreciated the larger parachutes as tents. They set up a seventy-foot Jeep parachute as a headquarters tent. Special Air Services trooper Wellsted described their construction: from a pole run horizontally through two trees, about five meters off the ground, they hung two parachutes, one inside the other. The material was then stretched tight and pegged with rigging lines, so the edges were slightly off the ground. The outer material, usually green or khaki for camouflage, served as rain-break, but was not waterproof. The inner parachute served as a second protection against the rain. A layer of forest ferns was scattered on the floor, and a third parachute laid on it. Parachute cords strung across wood frames made a mattress, and with a layer of moss and a parachute lining, sleeping bag on top, they called it comfortable.[21]

So after the Chateau de Vermot burned, Prochiantz turned to Louis Aubin (pseudonym Lafleur) and the Bernard maquis for help setting up a new infirmary. Aubin chose a spot near the kitchen and the mess hall, had a few trees cut down, leveled the ground, and raised a parachute tent. Lighting was provided by car headlights rigged to a battery, instruments boiled in a pot over a campfire. "Our operating room, while basic, was under a large white parachute, both pleasant and functional," Prochiantz wrote. It was set up just in time for SAS trooper Eric Adamson, whose Jeep overturned on July 4 on a rutted forest road, crushing his pelvis. It took twenty-four hours to get him to Prochiantz, who noted a double vertical fracture of the pelvis with accompanying internal damage. The surgeon went to work under the parachute tent, using a sterilized bicycle-pump tube as catheter. Two months later, they were able to send Adamson back to England on an airplane, and he recovered. In 1988, he wrote to Prochiantz to thank him "and all the other maquisards who were so kind to me, and took risks on my behalf. I watch rugby on television, and am always pleased to see France win."[22]

The Bernard camp was becoming a central command of sorts, as they were able to run a telephone line from it to a tiny abandoned train station at Coeuzon, outside Ouroux, and connect to the national network. The old station served as guardpost for the main entrance to the Bernard camp. In communications, the local telephone operator helped the guerrillas, as did two local residents fluent in German who listened in on German conversations and translated information about troop movements for the guerrillas. And the local postal carrier provided mail service to the camp. All it lacked was electricity and plumbing.

It would seem that the Germans could find the camp without too much trouble, but the SAS troopers noted that they kept off the back roads of the Morvan for fear of ambush. The unofficial split was that national roads were for the Germans; the departmental roads for the maquisards. Wellsted recounted a clash that occurred in mid-July when a German car got lost and came upon a maquisard car in the town of Ouroux. Each realized at the same moment that the other was the enemy and opened fire. Two maquis were wounded, and the Germans were killed except the driver, who had jumped into a roadside ditch and did not emerge until the maquisards were gone. Shot in the leg, he went to the village café for help. The café owner called the SAS, who came to take him prisoner, and as he recovered, they discovered he was not a Nazi and was opposed to the war. He became helpful around the camp, translating documents taken from a Gestapo car the maquis ambushed, for example.[23]

But all the camps were not as well protected by their neighbors. At Chaumard, twenty kilometers southwest of the Bernard camp, a new group of more than 160 young men had set up in early July. The number of guerrilla camps across the country was multiplying by midsummer as more and more men saw the maquis as a way to help fight in advance of a French army to join. The Chaumard group was infiltrated by a double agent and his teenage son, come to spy on them for the Germans. One night they took one of the camp's motorcycles and slipped out. Just before dawn on July 31, German soldiers surrounded the camp and blasted its wood-plank cabins with machine guns, killing twenty-two maquisards and taking four prisoner. A handful of men escaped, including one with a broken leg, hiking for ten hours to the next camp to find aid. The survivors were taken into the Bernard group, who went looking for and caught the traitors. They locked the father and son in the basement of the Coeuzon train station and held a forest trial, with Louis Aubin, some Bernard maquisards, and some SAS troopers as judge and jury. Hubert Cloix, a young business-school student who kept a journal of his time in the forest, wrote that the guerrillas were not seeking revenge. "The tribunal tried to save them, but they declared without shame that they wanted to escape and rejoin the Germans again. Given the declarations of the suspects, the tribunal wisely decided to condemn them to death. This extreme measure was justified by the security of the maquis and the Resistants," Cloix wrote.[24]

Cloix had joined a subcamp of the Bernard maquis led by Lt. André Guyot, a graduate of the Saint-Cyr military academy who had been recruited into the Vengeance network by Dr. Victor Dupont. Guyot had wanted to join the Free French in North Africa, but Dupont talked him into staying to fight from France. His guerrilla group was augmented by some local gendarmes who took to the forest in July. Guyot brought his military training and discipline to bear on the young recruits, beginning each morning with a flag-raising ceremony and spending hours a day training them in tactics, strategy, and protocol. Seven of his thirty men had worked with the Vengeance Resistance network, founded by Drs. Dupont, Wetterwald, and Chanel. Chanel had been arrested and deported in 1942; Dupont in 1943 and Wetterwald in January 1944. To avoid arrest themselves as the network crumbled, many of Vengeance's operatives moved to the maquis. André Guyot was happy to see them. On France's national day, July 14, 1944, about 150 guerrillas from various camps gathered to sing the national anthem around the flagpole. "[It was] a Marseillaise sung under the trees, facing the tri-colored French flag. Lt. André gave a short speech to castigate the enemy oppressing the country and to express the hope that, by our actions, the Nation would be liberated," Cloix wrote. "The lieutenant's speech, the raising of the colors, the singing of the Marseillaise, created a space of liberty counter to the constraints of the Occupation. What emotion to feel free and French! What happiness to feel capable of fighting for the Country!"[25]

The cooks made a special lunch of roasted chicken and potatoes for the occasion. Cherries were ripe on the trees, and the men went out and picked enough for everyone, no doubt singing the old song from a previous war *Le temps des cérises,* about a short time of happiness to be kept as a dear memory when heartbreak and loss follow. Shortly afterward, the National Resistance liaison, André Rondenay, left the Morvan to return to Paris and fell into a traitor's trap. He and four companions were arrested by the Gestapo, and after two weeks of interrogation, taken to the edge of a forest and shot. He was not quite thirty years old.

From Paris, the Committee of Medical Resistance weighed in with a set of guidelines for doctors working with the guerrillas. Prochiantz would have thrown them right back if he could have. Rule no. 1: "Don't establish a fixed clinic or hospital." Rule no. 2: "Don't use busy hospitals or clinics in major cities," find a more discreet facility and bring your own supplies. Rule no. 3: "Don't operate in the open air, in a forest, or in a rustic refuge. It's a romantic and heroic last resort, but if the wound is serious, one isn't doing real surgery."[26] It went on for several pages. Prochiantz noted that he had broken every one of the rules, but that the Germans did not capture a single one of his patients. During his three months in the forest, he carried out ninety-eight operations and saw twelve of his patients die. "The profession of surgeon to the guerrillas, like that of a maquisard, is learned in doing, in combat, and not by reading an official bulletin sent out after the fact."[27] Years later, he credited the purity of the forest air for patients' healthy healing despite the nonsterile conditions of operations. Other doctors among the Morvan maquis included Dr. Henri Smilovici, a Jewish Romanian who had immigrated to France in 1930, and Dr. Pierre Fouilloux, a local resident who had just completed his fourth year of medical studies in 1944.

In early August the Camille maquisard camp came under both air and ground attack by the Germans, but the SAS had a heavy six-pound antitank gun and managed to wipe out three enemy machine-gun positions and a mortar launcher. When the Germans persisted and forced the troopers and guerrillas to flee, they camouflaged the gun under some brush before they ran. Once the Germans had left, they got some farmers to bring an ox team to move it. The SAS were carrying out sabotage missions on the train tracks and industrial targets around the area, working with twenty-four-year-old Georges Brulé, a medical student and member of the Vengeance network. He also spoke English fluently. He and two companions had ridden their bicycles 250 kilometers from Paris to join the guerrillas. He worked with the SAS through the summer and after a parachute training course, joined their ranks in time to jump with the British forces in September 1944 at Arnhem in Operation Market Garden.

The Free French leaders in London had carved France up into regions, with the Morvan maquisards composing part of the larger operations in Burgundy's Region D. Directing the region was a young doctor, Claude Monod, son of the renowned surgeon Robert Monod, who was working in Paris with the Committee of Medical Resistance. Claude Monod was twenty-eight, a medical resident at Saint-Louis Hospital and member of the *Défense de la France* network when he was sent to Burgundy in June 1944. His initial mission was to sabotage and delay any German traffic going to defend against the Allied landings in Normandy; his later mission was to block German troop retreats eastward. Monod reported to London on August 6 that thus far, the maquisards and SAS had managed to cut 216 railroad lines and destroy twenty bridges, leading to twenty-six train derailments causing destruction of 465 wagons and fifty engines. They had cut fifty-four high-wire electric lines and all telephone lines. A total of 400 enemy soldiers had been killed and fifty taken prisoner.[28] A month later, the figures had grown to 350 rail lines, 615 wagons, and 75 engines destroyed, bringing an estimated 3,274 hours of delay to German convoys. The pressure on the occupier was mounting rapidly. The first week of September saw General George S. Patton's US Third Army arrive in the Marne, just north of Burgundy, while General Jean de Lattre de Tassigny's French First Army took Lyon, to the south. The Morvan sat in the middle of the squeeze, trying to keep the flow of information going to both, and to coordinate the thousands of maquisards in the fight. Monod wrote to London in his September report that the maquisards' role at that point was more vital to morale than to strategy: "Anyone who has lived with the maquisards for even a few days, it is impossible not to be struck by the fervor, the enthusiasm, the fighting spirit of the men," Monod wrote. "Despite the hard life, due to a lack of cantonments and a dearth of clothing, despite the insufficiency of a framework of instruction, there was no rebellion, no indiscipline. . . . These men have given their country the best of themselves."[29]

About half the guerrillas joined the Free French Army in September, including the majority of the Bernard group, creating the quickly dubbed Bernard Battalion. Monod joined the First Army as a lieutenant colonel and requested a posting to the 4th Régiment de Tirailleurs Marocains, which was expected to be first French artillery unit to cross the Rhine River. He crossed the Rhine, dividing France from Germany, on Easter Sunday, April 1, 1945, and led his troops through several German villages with no resistance, until he reached Graben. There, he was shot by a sniper while setting up machine-gun positions at the edge of the forest. A fellow soldier asked if he should bandage him, and Monod said there was no point, given his wound. He was a doctor. He knew he was going to die.

A month previously, Monod had written to his commanding general about returning to Burgundy to wrap up some final details. "And then it is over. Region D and the FFI [Forces françaises de l'intérieur) will become just a memory. It is only a slice of life that will crumble into the debris of the past. A bit of life that was brutal, passionate, but pure and beautiful, because at the end of the story was the risk of death. Our virtue, General, was to put into parallel the sense of duty and the fear of death, and to have chosen between the two. In that, we had the occasion once in our lives to have a notion of the absolute."[30]

In the forest of the Morvan, not far from the old Bernard camp, is a tiny cemetery bearing the graves of twenty-two maquisards and seven SAS who were killed that summer, along with the ashes of companions who died later and asked to join them. Beech and pine trees tower overhead in the constant play between growth and decay, the rich earth is furrowed by wild boars around the site, but alongside the graves, there is only peace. Their war is over.

9

AN AMERICAN DOCTOR
PITCHES IN

Most Americans left Paris during the first year of German occupation, believing it was just a matter of time before the United States entered the war. After it did declare war in December 1941, about five hundred Americans who had stayed behind were interned at Compiègne and held prisoner until 1944, while others were allowed their liberty due to age or professional considerations. American institutions in France also were under threat, and by 1941, almost all had either closed or taken French cover in order to remain in operation. The American Hospital of Paris was placed under the aegis of the French Red Cross, the American Library of Paris became a subsidiary of the French Information Center in New York, and the American Church on the quai d'Orsay joined the Protestant Reformed Church of France. Only the American Cathedral of the Holy Trinity, the Episcopal church on avenue George V, was left unprotected, and in August 1942 was taken over by the German Wehrmacht as its place of worship.

Of these establishments, the American Hospital was in the most tenuous position. The board of governors, before leaving for the United States, named as managing governor retired general Aldebert de Chambrun. Chambrun, seventy years old in 1942, had a sterling WWI record and a long history of association with American business and culture. He was president of the National City Bank branch in Paris from 1934 to 1940, and had helped found the French Information Center in New York in 1935. He was a descendant of the Marquis de Lafayette and was married to Clara Longworth, an Ohio-born society maven and Shakespeare scholar. But perhaps the strongest qualification for him to lead the hospital through the shadows of the Occupation was the fact that his only son, René, a lawyer, was married to Josée Laval, daughter of the Vichy premier Pierre Laval. The Chambruns had solid connections to people with the power to protect. The hospital board of governors decided that it would not admit Germans for treatment and instead took on the care of interned British citizens and French prisoners of war who had been released. In return, the Germans allowed the hospital to continue operating independently.

Sumner Waldron Jackson, tall, square-jawed, taciturn and reserved in the manner of his Maine upbringing, became chief of medical staff at the American Hospital in 1940. As a practicing urologist and surgeon, he was far removed from the stone quarries where, at age fourteen, he had followed his father in breaking rock for a living. His path to France began in the First World War. After dropping out of school as a teenager, Jackson returned to work his way through undergraduate studies and graduate from Jefferson Medical College in Philadelphia in 1914, then completed his residency at Massachusetts General Hospital in Boston over the next two years. In fall 1916, he joined the Harvard University volunteer medical unit in France, and when the United States entered the war in November 1917, he served in the US Army Medical Corps in France.

That was where he met Charlotte "Toquette" Barrelet de Ricou, a Swiss-born, French-raised nurse, dark-haired, with a delicate face and big brown eyes. They were married in France in November 1917, and after the war, they moved to Philadelphia, where Jackson began a medical practice under the wing of an older, established doctor. Within two years they returned to France. Charlotte was miserable in Philadelphia, far from her family, homesick for her culture, unhappy to the point of illness. Their return to France meant Jackson would have to submit to French rules for foreign-born doctors in order to practice. First, he had to pass the high-school baccalaureate exam, and his French was faulty at best. They hired a French tutor, Clémence Bock, fluent in both French and English, to help him through it.

"I had agreed to undertake the literary part of this preparation, without believing that this American would persevere in his resolution, although his sister-in-law had told me, 'When Jack makes a decision he sticks to it, and always succeeds,'" Clémence Bock wrote in a memoir.[1] After eight months of hard work and study, Jackson nonetheless failed the exam. He went to Algeria (then part of France), where the testing was considered a bit less rig-

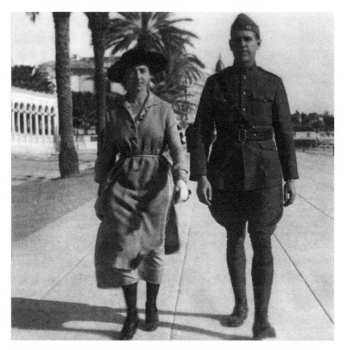

Dr. Sumner Jackson, chief medical officer at the American Hospital of Paris during the Occupation, and his wife, Charlotte, in a photo from the 1920s. American Hospital Archives.

orous, to retake it three months later, in October 1921. He passed. When he also succeeded at the medical school exam in 1925, they threw a big party to celebrate. He was finally on his way.

Jackson went directly on staff at the private, nonprofit American Hospital of Paris. A tiny early version of the hospital had been founded in 1909 to serve the growing American community in Paris. During the First World War, its governors had managed to set up and run a six-hundred-bed military hospital with private donations and volunteer medical staff, a tremendous effort that brought much gratitude and renown.[2] After the war, in 1926, the hospital opened a two-hundred-bed Memorial Wing, which served as the core facility for decades to come. That is where Jackson practiced, as well as at his private office in the family apartment at 11 avenue Foch. He never was entirely comfortable in French, and did not work in French hospitals.

In 1928, the Jacksons had a son, whom they named Phillip. They spent holidays at Charlotte's family lakeside home at Enghien, twenty-three kilometers north of Paris, sailing and playing tennis and being outdoors. Life was good. Jackson drove a 5-hp Citroën Type C for a few years, and then upgraded to a fancy Amilcar. When France began to feel the effects of the global Depression around 1930 and many Americans returned home, Jackson found his patient roster declining; he was less busy than he would have liked. But he and Phillip would go out on the boat on Lake Enghien, swimming and rowing, and to boxing matches. When Phillip's academic achievements were not what his father hoped, his mother mediated the disputes.[3]

And then came the second war. Jackson and a few other American doctors at the American Hospital stayed through the collapse and surrender in June 1940, as recounted in chapter 1. Dr. Edmund Gros, the hospital's seventy-three-year-old chief of staff, had a stroke and returned to the United States in October. Dr. Morris B. Sanders, an anesthesiologist who had done his residency at Massachusetts General with Jackson, and Dr. Daniel Hally-Smith, a surgeon-dentist with a practice at Place Vendôme since 1912, remained in Paris. Jackson and Charlotte discussed returning to the States, but Charlotte was strongly opposed. They stayed, and watched conditions under the Occupation become increasingly difficult.

Dr. Jackson was the only American left on the hospital governing committee when Aldebert de Chambrun was named managing editor. General de Chambrun would later refer to Jackson as "our greatly beloved chief of staff."[4] Morris Sanders wrote that before the war, Jackson had a twofold mission at the hospital: providing care to the resident American community and visitors in English and at a level they would find at home, and showcasing American medical and surgical techniques to European doctors. Sanders joined Jackson at the hospital in 1928, and he became a resident surgeon and anesthesiologist in 1932.

When the United States entered the war, Sanders and Hally-Smith were rounded up by German police and taken to the internment camp at Compiègne. Jackson, inexplicably, was not. General de Chambrun wrote to the German command and urged the doctors' release. The authorities agreed, if Sanders would agree to help German doctors with anesthesia for operations if needed. Hally-Smith, sixty-one years old, was released due to his age. It wasn't until September 1942 that Jackson was picked up by the police, along with four hundred other US citizens, and sent to Compiègne. Again, Chambrun intervened, and Jackson was released. He was busy at the hospital, which had been contracted by the Red Cross to care for hundreds of American and British military prisoners of war who fell ill in the internment camps.

Before the war, many prominent French doctors also consulted at the American Hospital, including Théodore Alajouanine, André Cain, Mathieu-Pierre Weil, Jean-Louis Deschamps, and Robert Debré. There was a certain amount of interaction between the French and American medical communities, much of it guided by research exchanges at organizations such as the Rockefeller Institute for Medical Research in New York. Some doctors who consulted at the American Hospital were deeply involved in the Resistance, such as André Ravina. But there is no evidence the hospital's staff carried out actions on the premises. Just across the rue du Chateau from the hospital stood the Feldgendarmerie, a German Army police headquarters, with the Feldkommandantur Paris-West (military field command station) and the Gestapo around the corner on boulevard Victor Hugo. Neuilly-sur-Seine counted four thousand billeted German troops among its population of 57,000 residents. The American Hospital, whatever the sympathies of its staff, was surrounded.

Individually, however, there was more room for careful action. In July 1943, a friend learned that young Phillip was going to visit family friends near the Atlantic coastal town of Saint Nazaire, where the Germans had a submarine base. Would he take some photographs of the base, covertly? He discussed it with his parents, and they agreed that he could. The friend gave him a small camera and showed him how to use it. In a videotaped interview years later, he dismissed the errand as "foolhardy" and "an exaggerated risk" that he did not measure at his age. "There was nothing heroic about it, it was childish recklessness."[5] Yet when he spoke of it, he smiled just a bit. Those were hard years; his successful mission no doubt retained a lasting glow of pride.

Despite the risk, another Resistance network approached Dr. Jackson at the hospital. Gladys Marchal, a hospital telephone operator and agent for the group *Ceux de la Libération,* brought an American airman to Dr. Jackson's office one afternoon in August 1943. The airman, Joseph Manos, a nineteen-year-old tail gunner from New York City, had been on a bombing run over northeastern France when his plane was hit by artillery fire. He backed out of the tail hatch and pulled the cord on his parachute at sixteen thousand feet, watching his plane go down in flames and explode upon impact. He thought he saw some other parachutes go out, but he couldn't be sure.[6]

Manos landed in a beet field, hid his parachute and life vest, and started moving toward a village he had seen from the air. Two young Frenchmen saw him on the road and warned him that a German soldier was approaching. Manos dove into a wheat field to hide. The young men followed him and then drove him in a truck to a home in Bondy, a northeastern suburb of Paris, and gave him civilian clothes. They said they would get him to Spain. They handed him over to a contact in Charenton, a suburb a few kilometers south. He stayed with a family there for a month. That was where Gladys Marchal picked him up and took him to the hospital. Would Dr. Jackson hide him in the hospital for a few days while they produced his false identity papers?

Jackson told Gladys Marchal it was "a crazy idea" to keep Manos at the hospital, according to Manos's later report.[7] Instead, he took him to his apartment. Jackson had given up his car in 1941, when fuel became scarce, and rode a bicycle, like the majority of Parisians. Manos rode the three miles on the handlebars. He stayed at the Jacksons' home for two days, and then Gladys Marchal picked him up and handed him over to network agent Gilbert Asselin. Manos spent three weeks in Asselin's apartment in Paris before being transferred south to Bordeaux, and eventually he hiked over the Pyrénées Mountains to Spain. He returned to England on November 30, after four months of clandestine living. Manos was lucky on many levels, to have survived the air attack as well as the many months of avoiding interaction with Germans or hostile French. One word out of his mouth and his American accent would have given him up. But he didn't know how lucky he was to have survived Gilbert Asselin. The next airman put into his care, along with the escape network helping him, was betrayed to the Gestapo. Two of the escape helpers died in concentration camps, and the airman was never heard of again. Years later, Asselin was reported by his comrades to have been a braggart, foolish, unstable. At the time, a fellow agent reported that Asselin had been showing off the Mauser submachine gun entrusted to him for security missions. No sooner had the network leaders confiscated the gun and booted Asselin out than the Gestapo burst in on a meeting and arrested them all. Asselin had led them there. He eventually was deported to Dachau himself, and served the SS guards as a trusty. "It is well-known that Asselin, to save his sweet face, gave it all up," a former comrade wrote in a report to the Interior Ministry official investigating Asselin's postwar claim of having been a Resistance agent.[8]

By the autumn of 1943, British and American air raids were intensifying, as the Allies tried to knock as much German infrastructure and resources out of commission as possible. Rumors of an Allied invasion proliferated, and the ranks of the Resistance grew. At the same time, the German and French police matched the expanding activity with increased investigations and surveillance. Pressure was rising on all sides.

The Jacksons' neighbor Francis Deloche de Noyelle, a twenty-two-year-old with a year of Resistance work already completed in eastern France, was looking for a Paris base. He liked the situation of the Jacksons' home, a ground-floor apartment on a corner, with two entrances, one on avenue Foch, the other on rue Traktir, down the street from his parents' apartment. Deloche de Noyelle asked Charlotte Jackson if the group could use their apartment as a letter drop and meeting place. Because Dr. Jackson had his office there, the comings and goings of strangers would not seem unusual, and the double entrances would make close surveillance more difficult. In January 1944, the Jacksons agreed to join Deloche de Noyelle's *Goélette* network. "In the end we decided to say yes, because it matched our opinions, our philosophy, and our desire for action," Phillip said.[9]

Their work was gathering information and transmitting it, with Charlotte the family's primary contact for the network. Dr. Jackson often stayed overnight at the hospital, and Phillip was sometimes sent to stay with friends or family when the apartment was needed for a meeting. People and papers began circulating in and out of the apartment with regularity. Even the maid, Louise Heile, knew what they were doing. Dr. Jackson was warned at least once by a friendly police officer to be careful, that he was being watched. "But he had such confidence in the speedy arrival of the Americans, and in final victory, that a new imprisonment did not frighten him, especially as his first experience had been so reassuring," Clémence Bock wrote, referring to his rapid release in 1942 from the Compiègne camp.[10] Her memoir recounted the events that followed.

A band of French militiamen, plain-clothes thugs who did the dirty work of the Gestapo, knocked at the Jacksons' door on the morning of May 25, 1944. Charlotte, quick-thinking, fixed them a drink and sent Louise on a fictitious errand, carrying a packet of compromising papers that should be removed from the apartment immediately. She and Phillip answered the men's questions politely, acting as though they had nothing to hide. Dr. Jackson was working at the hospital, so two of the militiamen went to get him. When he arrived, they began searching the apartment, turning it upside-down in a quest for incriminating evidence. They found nothing. Charlotte invited the militiamen for lunch, in an effort to be disarming. The men stayed, fending off telephone calls from the hospital for Dr. Jackson, and then spent the night at the apartment. The next morning, the men loaded the family into a car and drove them south to a prison near the town of Vichy. Louise wept, and stayed by the apartment window for days afterward to warn any Resistance agents away.

The Jacksons were interrogated by the Gestapo and then sent to the German military prison at Moulins. Apparently their names had been found on documents at the network's central office which had been seized the day before their arrest. Several agents had been summarily executed. In detention, Dr. Jackson and Phillip were held in the men's section; Charlotte in the women's. They caught a single glance of each other as they were being loaded into cars for the trip to Moulins. At the end of June, father and son were handcuffed together and put in a car for a twenty-hour road trip to the internment camp at Compiègne. Charlotte had been transferred to the women's prison at Fort Romainville, in an eastern suburb of Paris, earlier that month. Through the influence of the Swiss consul, Charlotte's sister was able to visit her there once, in early August. Charlotte reproached her for crying. On August 15, Charlotte was packed into a cattle car along with 2,200 other prisoners, on one of the last convoys to the concentration camps, leaving just ten days before Paris was liberated. The trip took six days, and when that ordeal ended at the gates of Ravensbrück concentration camp in Germany, another hell began, one that for Charlotte, would last eight long months.

Dr. Jackson and Phillip followed a similarly harsh path to the labor camp at Neuengamme, a prison complex of concrete, barbed-wire, and brutal SS guards. Dr. Jackson, now fifty-nine, was put to work in a welding shop, but in a matter of months, became a patient in the prison clinic with edema, or swelling in his legs, due to malnutrition. He began taking care of other patients in the clinic, and eventually he was allowed to work there instead. The camp clinic consisted of four barracks, but as at Buchenwald, self-appointed *kapos* grabbed positions as they liked, with no qualifications whatsoever. Charles-Julien Kaufmann, a French doctor imprisoned at Neuengamme, wrote that the clinic's "chief surgeon" was a truck driver, and no one was allowed to watch him operate. The camp had as many as three thousand patients at a time, with a supply of fifty aspirin per week. "Here medicine did not consist of healing, but only in preserving a slightly ill patient from a fatal decline. Beyond care, it was sleep and good treatment that our comrades needed most," Kaufmann wrote. "It was characteristic of all new entrants into the infirmary to start by sleeping for 48 hours straight."[11]

In the course of treating a prisoner's abscess, Jackson picked up an infection in his middle finger. There was little in the way of medical material or antiseptics; it got worse and worse. A Czech surgeon, a fellow prisoner, finally had to amputate it. Phillip, meanwhile, worked pushing wheelbarrows in the field and then got transferred to kitchen duty, a far better position during the cold winter months. He was one of twenty-eight cooks stirring thin rutabaga soup, sometimes from midnight to 4 a.m. At Neuengamme, nearly half the 100,000 prisoners died, of disease, malnutrition, overwork, or execution. By spring, rumors of the approach of Allied troops brought a thaw of optimism, but on April 21 the camp was evacuated, the prisoners put on trains for the northern port of Lübeck, on the Baltic Sea. Ten days later, told they would be sent to Sweden, they were boarded onto three ships that motored out and anchored in the bay of Neustadt. Sumner and Phillip Jackson were on the *Thielbeck,* along with two thousand other prisoners crammed into the hold, many of them ill. Dr. Kaufmann, on the second ship, the *Cap Arcona,* wrote that they set up a clinic in the lowest level of the ship and nursed the ill as best they could, but that they were given neither food nor water for eight days. Prisoners were dying of hunger, and then a typhus epidemic erupted.

Swedish diplomat Folke Bernadotte, working through the Swedish Red Cross, had been negotiating prisoner releases with the Germans. In April 1945, he met with SS Chief Heinrich Himmler, architect of the genocide, whom Bernadotte described as becoming more and more nervous as the Allies drew near. Himmler agreed to free some European and American prisoners from Neuengamme, which Bernadotte wrote "was believed to be one of the worst."[12] Among the Neuengamme camp prisoners was Michel Hollard, a French resistant whose covert report on the construction of German rocket-launch pads in northern France had allowed the British to destroy them. A postwar book on his exploits was titled *The Man Who Saved London.* As the released group was gathering, Hollard saw Dr. Jackson on the quay by the train wagons they were using for patient care, and urged him to join them. As an American, he could walk away. "Jackson made no answer but, raising his arm wearily, pointed to the prostrate figures covering the floor of the wagon. They were the bodies of his dying patients," Hollard recounted in his book.[13] Jackson remained behind.

Bernadotte also had arranged for some women to be freed from Ravensbrück and its associated labor camps. Charlotte Jackson was one of five women with American citizenship who were released on April 28 and taken to Mälmo, Sweden, where they were treated for the illnesses they had suffered and the damage prolonged malnutrition had caused. Charlotte, at fifty-five, had lost most of her teeth. She had no idea what had happened to her husband and son, if they were alive, or where they might be. As she recovered in Sweden, Dr. Jackson and his son were packed into the hold of the *Thielbeck*. While his father looked after the ill among them, Phillip climbed a narrow iron ladder up to the top deck for some air. It was the middle of the afternoon on May 3. He saw a squadron of British Hawker Typhoon planes buzzing overhead, and then suddenly the rockets rained down. The ship, shattered, began sinking rapidly into the bay. Phillip stripped down, looking desperately for his father to emerge on deck. He did not, and with the ship sliding deeper, Phillip plunged into the icy water.

"I am a very good swimmer and was able to board one of the salvage boats the Germans had lowered," he wrote in a report five days later. "I was saved before they knew we were prisoners. When they did know, they saved their sailors and soldiers only and let drown over a thousand prisoners who were swimming."[14]

As they reached the shore, SS troops opened fire on them, but Phillip scrambled to safety. He never saw his father again. He wrote that one of the other French prisoners told him he had seen Dr. Jackson swimming, holding onto a plank, in trouble. Only about five hundred men (among them Dr. Kaufmann) survived, of the seven thousand prisoners on the three ships. The British Royal Air Force had believed the ships carried escaping Nazi troops and had warned their captains to return to dock. The SS officers ordered the *Thielbeck* and *Cap Arcona* to remain in the bay, and while the third ship, the *Athen,* did return, it also was bombed. Red Cross officials had informed the British command that there were prisoners on the ships in Neustadt Bay, but the information was not passed on to the RAF 2nd Tactical group, tasked with blocking Nazi leaders from escaping into Norway. Watching from the quay in horror were British ground troops just arriving at Lübeck and several hundred prisoners who had been taken off the *Athen.*

Among them was Simon Lubicz, the doctor who had worked at Compiègne and at Auschwitz. He and the others were taken into care by the Swedish Red Cross and evacuated from Germany.

Phillip Jackson immediately joined the British Army as an interpreter for a medical unit. He thought his mother was dead; it wasn't until weeks later that he learned she had survived. The following year, he testified in the war crimes trial of fourteen SS guards from the Neuengamme camp who were arrested by the British. Eleven of the men were sentenced to death by hanging. Postwar, both Phillip and his mother were named Chevaliers in the Legion of Honor; all three Jacksons were awarded a Croix de Guerre, the highest French military honor. Paul Kinderfreund, who was the Jacksons' Resistance supervisor in *Goélette,* noted on a report of their work: "Everything was given to the Allied cause with total selflessness, constant devotion and superb courage, the greatest of services."[15]

The American Hospital of Paris, with 250 beds and 250 employees, managed to stay open throughout the Occupation, despite the fact that most of the expatriate population, its patient base, was gone. General de Chambrun and the board feared that if the hospital was not running at capacity, it would be requisitioned by the Germans. Chambrun did have to send annual financial reports to the German military command detailing the hospital's income and expenses, and there were occasional disagreements over whether a prisoner was fit to return to an internment camp. Doctors tried to prolong the prisoners' hospital stays as long as they could. Treatment of interned Americans and British, paid by the respective governments through Red Cross organizations, provided a basic level of business and income.

Two French doctors, neither without controversy, contributed to the hospital staying afloat. Dr. Alexis Carrel had won a Nobel Prize in 1912 for developing techniques of vascular surgery, and his subsequent work in the First World War led to the first effective antiseptic against infection, saving untold numbers of lives. But in the late 1930s, his attention had shifted to race-based eugenics and parapsychology research. Carrel had set up the *Fondation Française pour l'Etude des Problèmes Humains* (French Foundation for the Study of Human Problems), funded by the Vichy government, to research ways of strengthening genetic inheritance in society, which he believed was degenerating. His theories aligned closely with Nazi ideas about racial hierarchy, and after the war he was accused of collaboration, but he died in November 1944 without trial.

During the First World War, Carrel had worked closely with the American Hospital, and he also had maintained a relationship with the Rockefeller Institute for Medical Research in New York, which had sponsored his earlier research. In 1942, he approached the hospital with a proposal to create a clinic to treat accidents occurring in the workplace. Carrel wanted to develop a standard of treatment and compensation for workers injured on the job, and proposed setting up a center for SNCF (national railway) workers at the hospital. Hospital surgeons André Lambling, Marcel Boppe, and Marc Iselin were among those who operated on injured railway workers, in a precursor to the field of occupational medicine that would emerge after the war. The SNCF paid the workers' medical costs, thus providing some support to the hospital during the Occupation. In 1943, the SNCF workers' center brought in 1.2 million FF ($4,200 at the black-market rate), nearly as much as the British government paid for its internee patients. Some further funding, 520,000 FF ($1,800), came from the French government for care of French prisoners of war sent from their camps.

Then came the arrival of Dr. René Leriche, the first president of the higher council of the Medical Order, whose inability to lift the ceiling on Jewish practitioners had brought criticism from one side, while the other side railed that he allowed Jews to practice at all. Leriche quit that post in December 1942 and became chief surgeon at the American Hospital. He had the problem of an outsider in France: he had studied and begun his career in Strasbourg, and with the war moved his practice to Lyon. Even with his appointment to the chair of medicine at the prestigious Collège of France and his reputation as a brilliant surgeon, no room was made for him in a Paris hospital. As he had visited the United States and had ties with top surgeons there, the American Hospital was a viable career alternative. Leriche was interested in the physiology of pain, one of the first doctors to investigate its causes and symptoms, especially in post-operative cases. He proposed setting up a clinic to conduct scientific studies of pain at the hospital, and the board agreed.

General de Chambrun announced to the Germans in May 1944 that Dr. Leriche's research laboratory on pain had required some expense on the part of the hospital and was not expected to earn back its investment immediately. "The object of this institution being to render service to liberated war wounded and to the surgical and medical clientele and to end the year without a deficit, this goal has been reached despite all the difficulties of the moment, thanks to the devotion of the personnel and to healthy management," Chambrun wrote in his report.[16] While his description of the pain clinic's effect on hospital finances was negative in his report to the Germans and positive in his report to the hospital board, his motivation for each position can be surmised. The two research centers, treating pain and work accidents, were keeping the hospital's beds full. Like most of France, the hospital was doing its best to maintain its activity and its identity through the treacherous terrain of the Occupation. While Carrel and Leriche had much to recommend them in terms of medicine, the reputations of both were tainted by their political connections. The hospital board took advantage of being a "foreign" hospital to sidestep the politics in favor of the medicine. It was an effective tactic, and the hospital's reputation for neutrality stood firm. In its plans for medical care during the liberation campaign, the Resistance Medical Committee listed the American Hospital in Neuilly as a place where injured rebels could safely be taken for treatment.

After Paris was liberated, in an echo of WWI, the US Army took over the American Hospital, turning it into the US 365th Station Hospital and assigning it primary care for American military officers, civilians of officer status, and all women military personnel in the Paris region. The Army hired twenty of the hospital's staff nurses and twenty support and maintenance personnel during the time it ran the hospital. It housed nearly half the enlisted personnel in the former Feldgendarmerie across the street. Only once during its eighteen-month stint as a military hospital did it treat battle casualties; it took in a hundred soldiers injured in the Battle of the Bulge in December 1944. Along with medical care, the Army set up sports and recreation activities for patients and staff, including tennis and horseshoe pitching; opened a soda fountain and ice-cream bar, and showed movies three nights a week. In March 1946, the hospital was returned to its civilian administrators. The Army left behind a gift: the refrigerator it had installed to store the new miracle drug, penicillin.[17]

10

LIBERATION AT LAST

After the D-Day landings beginning June 6, 1944, it took the Allied armies seventy-five days to break out of Normandy and push the bulwark of German troops there into an eastward retreat. By mid-August tension in Paris was running high. Where were the Americans? When would they liberate the capital? Some in the Resistance did not want to wait, believing they could end the German Occupation themselves and reap the political reward for having done so. With sixteen major Resistance groups united in the Conseil National de la Résistance (National Council of Resistance), they represented a panoply of political creeds, most of them keeping a calculating eye on the postwar political horizon.

The doctors' Resistance committee met on August 10 at the spacious Paris apartment of Dr. Victor Veau, a seventy-two-year-old surgeon and WWI veteran, who kept a detailed diary of the tumultuous days of August. "The meeting was fairly agitated—we heard some shouting," he wrote.[1] In attendance were Louis Pasteur Vallery-Radot, Paul Milliez, Robert Merle d'Aubigné, Thérèse Bertrand-Fontaine, Robert Debré, Raymond Leibovici, and Hector Descomps. The latter three represented the left-leaning National Front and were frequently at odds with some more conservative members. Their goal was the same, but their ideas of how to achieve it did not always coincide.

Robert Debré and Elisabeth de La Bourdonnaye had moved back from the suburbs to her apartment on the rue de Varenne in August to be at hand for the action. Debré was in charge of Resistance medical services for the city of Paris, working with FFI leader Henri Rol-Tanguy, who directed operations from his cellar communications headquarters at Place Denfert-Rochereau (today the city of Paris's Musée de la Libération).

Meanwhile, Robert Merle d'Aubigné had set up his mobile surgical teams, along with medical material stockpiles, in the Seine-et-Oise department of suburbs surrounding Paris. In the capital, material had been hidden mainly at the Institut Pasteur. They had amassed 25 kilograms of potassium permanganate, 20,000 glass vials of morphine, 20,000 bandages, and 20,000 doses of antitetanus serum. In departments farther from the capital, they gathered 3,000 bandages, 3,000 doses of anti-tetanus serum, and 25 kilograms of powdered sulfonamides, the antibiotic of the time. Robert Monod had organized supplies for the northern suburbs of the Oise department. The most difficult to stock were surgical instruments and material. While some material had been parachuted in from London and transported to safe storage by agents in the postal service, other items had to be purchased. None of it was easily done. As late as March 1944, when the country was running desperately short of medical material, French authorities who inadvertently discovered a stockpile alerted the Vichy government—which immediately turned it over to the Germans. The doctors fumed.

The Resistance Medical Committee had begun drafting instructions in March, well before the Allied landings, for medical care during insurrection fighting in the capital. The idea was to have mobile teams ready and equipped to go to the injured, anticipating that transportation would be shut down and access to hospitals difficult. "The mobile surgical teams are being created to remedy as much as possible the impossibility of evacuation. Their role consists in practicing in the full center of operations, with rudimentary means, surgery of extreme urgency, which will keep those with relatively light wounds from succumbing due to lack of care," the instructions explained.[2]

Teams should consist of a young surgeon, unencumbered by regular hospital duties, an assistant doctor, an anesthetist, and a nurse. Instructions directed: recruit stretcher bearers where you need them, ask for linens and pots in which to sterilize instruments from nearby residents, and raid local pharmacies for whatever you need. Each team should carry in a backpack equipment that included scalpels, clamps, curettes, needles and catgut, amputation saw, bandages, and masks, as well as anesthetic, antiseptic, and antibiotic products in various forms. And don't forget a flashlight.

With all the members of the doctors' committee living clandestinely by 1944, they met in train stations and churches, eating meals with friends at their homes rather than in restaurants. Victor Veau's apartment off the Place Saint Augustin in the Eighth Arrondissement became a base of sorts. His cook, identified only as Camille, regularly prepared lunches and dinners for PVR and his wife Jacqueline and various other members of the medical resistance. Veau, a pioneer and specialist in repairing cleft palates, reported that by August 15, cooking gas had been cut to mealtimes, electricity was on for an hour at noon and then from 10 p.m. to 5 a.m.; the Metro had ceased to run and the stores were closed. While his neighborhood bakery stayed open, the line was long and the bread ersatz, when available. But, he noted with delight, the Germans were packing up and leaving town.

Their only source of outside information came from the radio, mainly the BBC from London. While it did a herculean job of informing the cloistered French how the Allied fighting was going, it was only as good as its sources, and its reporters were censored by the armies. On August 19, Veau noted that according to news reports, the Americans were at Versailles, just twenty kilometers west of Paris. They were not. Rumor and misinformation swirled into the churn of trepidation, sometimes leading to tragedy. A friend told Veau that on August 15, a group had gathered at the Porte d'Orléans, a southern entrance to the city, believing the Americans were going to arrive at any moment. A random gunshot was fired. "The Germans took the opportunity to machine-gun the crowd. Many deaths," Veau noted.

Among the top German commanders who left town was Aloïs Brunner, the sadistic commander of the Drancy internment camp. He took with him, on August 17, fifty-one Jewish prisoners from Drancy, who joined 1,249 prisoners from Compiègne to constitute the last convoy of deportees to Buchenwald. With French train workers on strike and tracks sabotaged around much of the Paris area, the deportees were driven by truck to an eastern forest and packed into cattle cars for the rest of the trip. Hours before, Swedish consul Raoul Nordling had negotiated an agreement with the Paris-based Wehrmacht command to turn all prisoners and camps over to the Red Cross, but not all the Nazis were in agreement. Nordling tried twice to stop the train; twice he failed. Brunner slipped away in Germany, avoiding arrest after the war and living unrepentant to the age of eighty-nine in Syria, believed to have been a consultant to the government's interrogation units there. Before leaving, Brunner turned the Drancy camp over to a

Wehrmacht unit which, in line with its agreement, then asked Nordling to take responsibility. Nordling brought a young Red Cross social worker, Annette Monod, to Drancy and put her in charge of its remaining 1,500 prisoners. Monod had worked briefly at the camp in 1941, and at several other internment camps since, and judged with a keen eye what needed to be done. She gathered the camp leaders and told them flatly that the Germans still held Paris. "*Voilà,* you are free, you can leave if you like, but—there is a great risk," she recounted saying in an interview years later. "They would have been killed."[3]

The SS and police guards at Rothschild Hospital also abandoned their post on August 18, the day after Brunner fled. Robert Debré sent a member of the Resistance Medical Committee to take charge, and Rothschild became one of the main hospitals for treating those injured in the early insurrection. A squad of Resistance fighters also arrived to defend it from pro-German militia, who had taken up positions in the neighboring Picpus Cemetery, resting place of the Marquis de Lafayette, and fired on the hospital. Their days were numbered.

As the enticing vision of liberation drew closer, Resistance members clashed in heated argument: was it the moment for insurrection? The FFI and its communist union leader Rol-Tanguy pushed for an uprising. On August 19, the FFI and striking police officers took possession of the Préfecture de Police headquarters in Paris, and Resistance agents began carrying out guerrilla strikes on German troops patrolling the capital. German tanks returned their pistol fire with mortar shells, an exchange that did not bode well for the city or for the Resistance, and a cease-fire was rapidly arranged. The center-right Gaullist Resistance, supporting the truce, argued that with only two to three thousand active agents in the city, and not all of them armed, they did not have enough firepower to sustain an offensive. An uprising at this moment would lead to a massacre. Paris was cut off, the trains on strike, the Metro closed, German barricades blocking city exits. The capital was in a tense and terribly fragile state. Most FFI combatants, however, refused to honor the truce and continued their attacks. Resistance Medical Committee members met at 5:30 p.m. that day at Dr. Veau's apartment. Leftist members opposed the truce, rightist members supported it, but their antagonism was ebbing. "The meeting lasted two hours, less stormy than usual," Veau noted in his diary. "They left with a smile."

Then the Resistance learned that Vichy premier Pierre Laval planned to return to Paris, summon the National Assembly, and ensure that Vichy-friendly representatives were seated. Marshal Pétain would retire, the Assembly would approve a similar figurehead, and power would remain in the same hands—most of all, out of the reach of the Free French. The old Vichy government would pretend to have always been on the side of the French people, and for the sake of peace, many would be ready to accept that prevarication. It was a fiendishly clever plan, and it kept Dr. Robert Monod awake all night with worry. By the time the sun came up on August 20, Monod had found a possible solution and, first thing, rang Robert Debré. They met, and Debré agreed: if they could persuade the American troops, now reportedly just sixty kilometers west of Paris, to change their plans and hurry to the capital, it would flip the advantage to the Resistance. Debré contacted Rol-Tanguy, who sent a messenger with instructions to ask the Americans only for a parachute drop of weapons and munitions. The FFI could handle the rest, he believed.

Dr. Monod filled up the tank of his Peugeot 202 at a clandestine fuel depot and picked up the messenger, Roger Cocteau, pseudonym Commandant Gallois, a former army officer who was one of the leaders of the *Ceux de la Libération* Resistance group. In April 1944, he had taken over as military director for the Paris area, serving as Rol-Tanguy's right-hand man. He also was fluent in English. With Monod's *Ausweis* travel pass on the windshield, they drove west out of the city, concocting a story about going to check on children in a suburban TB sanatorium. They were stopped several times and made to turn around by German troops, spending the night outside the western suburb of St. Nom-la-Bretèche, and in the morning Monod decided they should drive southward, where he had a Resistance cell contact and also thought the approach might be less guarded. Along the way, they talked at length about the situation, and Monod was frank: without an Allied approach, Paris was in great danger. It was not simply a question of getting more pistols to go up against German tanks. Cocteau agreed. Never mind his initial instructions, he would ask for a liberation operation. They discussed various approaches as the kilometers rolled by. "We were dying of hunger, we had had nothing to eat since lunch the day before, apart from some sugar cubes [Cocteau] had wisely brought, and we were falling asleep, after two consecutive nights on the go," Monod wrote in his memoir. "But there was not a minute to lose."[4] They finally stopped for lunch in a town about thirty kilometers south of Paris, and met up with the Resistance group there. The group agreed to take Cocteau on westward to Chartres, where a forward unit of American soldiers had arrived. Monod returned to Paris.

On August 20, after meeting with Monod, Robert Debré had joined PVR at Dr. Veau's apartment, watching the occasional passing car and motorcycle flying FFI banners, when they got a phone call from the dean of the Paris Medical School. He wanted to raise the French flag over the school, did they want to help? They most definitely did. Veau noted that they ran off "excited as children." Despite the rising violence in the streets, they managed to hoist the *bleu-blanc-rouge* over the boulevard Saint Germain. Their colors were flying again.

That same day, in Neuilly-sur-Seine, a group of some fifty FFI had tried to take over City Hall, killing seven German soldiers and drawing a severe response from the local SS and Wehrmacht units. Several Resistance fighters were killed and two dozen city employees taken prisoner, later exchanged for German prisoners. Courageous young people and students, unaware that the end-game moment was perhaps the most dangerous of all, were shot dead across the city. Veau was deeply worried. "We hear from very sure sources that the Allies will not be able to arrive for another 8 to 10 days," he wrote. "It will certainly be the annihilation of the FFI and the carnage of Paris."

Debré set up his medical command center in an underground office used by sewer workers just behind Val-de-Grace Hospital, and went to inspect emergency aid stations along the riverbank quays. As he reached Place St. Michel, where FFI agents hunkered behind a barricade, a truck with German soldiers drove through. An exchange of gunfire left dead and wounded in the street. Debré organized an impromptu treatment center in a café and called the nearest emergency station to send help. Then another German truck drove into the place, and a Frenchman leapt onto the running board to stop it. Shots rang out and he fell; the truck driver also was shot. Debré wrote that he ran out to help them: "The crowd shouted: 'Leave the dirty Boche, take care of the French!' Both soon were dead. The crowd abused the German's body. I had them both transported away."[5] With reports of injuries and fighting rolling in, Debré rode his bicycle from situation to situation. At Paris City Hall, he found French and German wounded inside, and the parvis in front of the building covered in broken window glass.

When he returned to Paris, Monod went straight to work at Laennec Hospital, where doctors operated on some two hundred people wounded

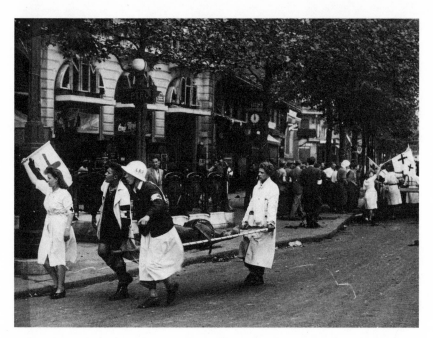

Red Cross workers on boulevard Saint Michel evacuating a wounded person as the uprising begins in August 1944. Copyright © Agence LAPI/LAPI/Roger-Viollet.

in the fighting, including a half-dozen Germans. He wrote that doctors and nurses at Cochin Hospital on the boulevard Port Royal, and at Hôtel Dieu Hospital on the Ile-de-la-Cité, were the busiest during those heated days. "In the heart of the battle, [we were] working without a break. Day and night, medical and nursing personnel, in a great gesture of patriotic solidarity, devoted themselves unreservedly."

The Resistance Medical Committee plan was working very well, he noted, with field stations in every neighborhood providing immediate first aid, and ambulances flying Red Cross flags making the rounds to pick up patients and take them to hospitals. It was dangerous work. He recalled seeing a young bicyclist shot in the back on the boulevard Saint Germain. They put her in his car and rushed her to the hospital, but she died.

"One of the more moving memories of that street combat was the sight in fire zones of those young women: unconcerned bicyclists in light dresses or nurses in white blouses, rushing between combatants, seemingly unaware of the danger," Monod wrote. "They were crazily courageous, to the shame of certain men who, as soon as the risk was over, showed up to quickly grab the best positions and push themselves to the front of the shower of rewards."[6]

Part of the Resistance plan included a letter to local doctors attaching them to army services as soon as insurrection began. "Paris risks, in a day, from one hour to another, to be plunged into bloody street fighting. We would not want any fresh weaknesses to remind us of the behavior of some in June 1940. We are certain you will do your duty with the greatest devotion."[7] The tone was acidly clear. At the same time, instructions called for immediate purging of Vichy medical officials. Plans dated May 1944 offered a letter formula for stripping officials of their posts, in the name of the Provisional Government of the French Republic, the name taken by the Free French administration somewhat in advance of the fact. The instructions emphasized that this "purification" was to be carried out on a strictly professional level.

PVR and Milliez, named by the National Council of Resistance as new health minister and chief of staff, were given approval on August 21 to take over the Health Ministry. Milliez rode over on his bicycle first. PVR was to meet him there, if a firefight raging outside Dr. Veau's window died down. Several young men in the street were killed, and then a German machine gun opened up, spraying the apartment and destroying the pharmacy one floor below. PVR hit the floor. When Milliez arrived at the ministry, he announced to the guard at the door that he had come to take possession in the name of the Resistance. The guard saluted and ushered him in to the chief of staff's office. "In plain view on the table were files of letters of denunciation, all signed by well-known doctors, likely the only letters that were kept. I knew the doctors they denounced, they were Jews, or married to Jews, or suspected of having friends who were Jews or English," he wrote. "Some of them were close friends of mine."[8]

Milliez threw the letters in a trash can and burned them all. Among them were letters from doctors who since had changed sides, at least one of whom was working with Milliez and PVR. Milliez felt it would be better to destroy them all than to allow for the possibility of revenge or blackmail down the road. PVR arrived, and the first thing he did was take down the portrait of Marshal Pétain. Ministry staff members, loyal to Pétain just moments before, measured the shift of power and duly applauded.

That same day, Annette Monod, a member of the extensive Protestant Monod clan and thus cousin to Robert Monod, released the last prisoner from the Drancy internment camp. She had spent three days working with the Drancy mayor's office and a Jewish welfare agency to get the prisoners equipped with identity papers, food, and a place to stay for those who no longer had a home. She had stayed in Brunner's old office, sleeping on a tablecloth in his bed as there were no clean sheets, eating chocolate she found stashed away. With the job finished, a Red Cross truck drove her back to the Red Cross office on rue de Berri, where she deposited the dossiers she had found in the camp administration office. She reported that the streets of Paris were deserted except for occasional squads of armed German soldiers, waiting and watching. Some twenty thousand German troops were still in the city, most of them holed up in defensible structures such as the Luxembourg Palace, the Hôtel des Invalides and the Lycée Montaigne.

On August 22, Dr. Bertrand-Fontaine returned to Paris from a trip to the provinces for the CMR. "She crossed German and American lines," Dr. Veau wrote. "A German soldier helped her carry her bicycle to cross the trenches of 'no-man's-land.'" He might not have done so had he known she was a Resistance agent. Also that day, they heard that the BBC reported that Paris was occupied—but by whom? "This is craziness. Or a mistake. Or politics," Veau wrote. With truth, the first casualty of war, down, they had only rumor, misinformation, and their own observations of a constantly shifting ground to go on, all to the occasional roar of artillery in the background. Debré learned that his younger son Olivier was seriously wounded by shrapnel near the Place de la République during an attack on a German army garrison. He was taken to Saint Antoine Hospital, and spent months recovering. The Medical Committee met again, in a tone of calm, at Veau's apartment, and in the August heat drank ten carafes of water. "I have run out of sherry and have no gas to make tea," he noted. It was a quiet night, no traffic or shooting. "Are they gone?"

The Paris Wehrmacht commander, General Dietrich von Choltitz, told Raoul Nordling that he believed Hitler was insane, but he had been ordered by the German high command to remain in place and to blow Paris sky-high with explosives if the Allies entered. At the same time, he wrote in a memoir, the lower-ranking officers, seeing their foothold disintegrate, were pushing hard to evacuate the city. "As always, interests of very different natures converged at the same point: I wanted to preserve my soldiers from any losses and the French were motivated to conserve their capital," Choltitz wrote.[9]

On Thursday, August 24, Robert Monod heard a rapidly spreading rumor that the Americans were at the Porte d'Orléans. He jumped in his car and drove down on the avenue, seeing crowds of people lining up on either side, heads turned south. But no Americans. He kept driving, and about five kilometers southwest, in the town of Clamart, he encountered the Free French Second Armored Division, led by General Leclerc. Cocteau's mission had succeeded.

Cocteau recounted that he had finally found a small unit of American soldiers, who took him at midnight to an officer who was not in uniform, and Cocteau didn't know who he was until later: General George S. Patton, commander of the US Third Army. Patton gave him a glass of Champagne, but turned down his plea for help, saying that Paris was not a military objective and that it would be a logistical nightmare to try to feed and protect its population. Nonetheless, he sent Cocteau by Jeep to a base outside the town of Laval, where he was presented to a panel of high-ranking Allied officers. Postwar, Cocteau said that since his first argument of urgent need had not worked, he switched to a new one. "France will never forgive America if it does not make an effort to save its city, which is already halfway liberated by its residents," Cocteau told them. "It was a big bluff."[10]

It worked. General Leclerc, arriving at Laval by plane from the Normandy town his troops had just cleared of Germans, was in "a black fury" over the fate of Paris, Cocteau said. Then General Omar Bradley, new commander of the Twelfth US Army Group, flew in and announced that it was on: Leclerc was authorized to take his Second Armored Division to the capital, backed up by the US Fourth Infantry Division. The generosity of the gesture would justify the logistical complications. Leclerc flew back to Sées in Normandy, signing the order to his troops at midnight. *En avant!* Two columns of tanks and other military vehicles raced some two hundred kilometers, through sporadic but significant fighting, to reach the gates of Paris on the night of August 24. Leclerc sent a reconnaissance unit, the Ninth Company (nicknamed *La Nueve* for its many Spanish Republican members), into the city, but waited for daylight to move the rest.

When he came upon French troops outside Paris, Monod felt a surge of emotion: "[It was] an unforgettable moment, anticipated hour after hour through four long and hard years of the Occupation. In the gathering dusk, among the scattered crowd lining this suburban street, the joy was fervent. One felt moved to tears by this first contact."[11]

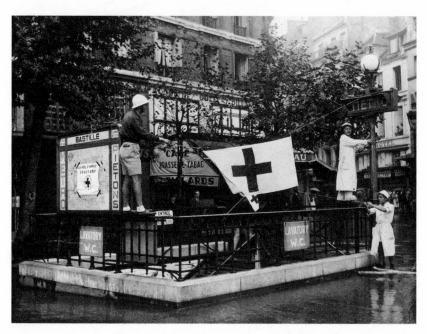

Red Cross workers setting up an aid station at Metro Bastille in Paris, August 1944.
Copyright © Service Historique de la Défense 2007 DE ZC 18/1 13099.

The following day, as French and American tanks, Jeeps, and other armored vehicles poured into Paris, the city erupted in exhilaration, makeshift flags fluttered from windows, women kissed every soldier they could reach, and children danced around the grinding tanks as though they were toys. "What an unforgettable spectacle! It is something to be seen," Veau wrote. "Civilians have no notion of war! Thousands of tanks and other cars are surrounded by an immense crowd, deliriously shouting and applauding." He noted the sea change from just the previous day. "It is hard to imagine that yesterday was the most horrifying terror. How can we pass so quickly to such a diametrically opposed state?"

But the war was not over, the city was not yet free, and some of the celebrants lost their lives. Many of the wounded were people watching from apartment windows, struck by random gunfire. Then, as troops gathered near the Arc de Triomphe, the echo of a shot fired prompted gunners to unload their automatic weapons into a nearby building. It happened to be the Health Ministry, where a group had gathered to observe. "Everyone was on the second floor and when the shooting began they ducked behind what they thought was a wall, but it was just a partition and was traversed by the bullets," Veau wrote. Norman Lewis, fifty-one, an American long resident in Paris who had been released recently from the Compiègne internment camp, was killed. A banker and president of the American Club, Lewis had brought an American flag to raise over the building. Two women also were wounded.

Taking a westerly approach, a Second Armored Division tactical group led by Colonel Jean Rémy rolled into Neuilly-sur-Seine, where the German army post (Feldkommandantur) across the street from the American Hospital was still fully staffed with six hundred armed men. The Gestapo headquarters down the street was run by the SS, and both units continued to defend their positions. The tanks of Rémy's Second Armored Naval Regiment drew enemy mortar fire, and casualties mounted.

At the American Hospital, Director Aldebert de Chambrun, fearing the worst, contacted the German army commander across the street and asked him to surrender. "After repeated colloquy with the German commander he became convinced that further resistance would only entail much bloodshed and the destruction of the Hospital; he consented to enter into negotiation with any regular force, either American or French," Chambrun wrote in a report to the hospital board.[12] "Thus the Hospital, in avoiding this battle, was saved from certain bombardment and possible destruction."

In exchange, for the first time in the war, the hospital took in and treated German patients. The Second Armored Division after-action report on the surrender did not mention Aldebert de Chambrun's role, but it did confirm that the German colonel surrendered and ordered his men, some still shooting from the rooftop of the Feldkommandantur, to lay down their arms. "Result of the operation: more than 800 prisoners, a thousand individual weapons, 10 tons of ammunition, mines and explosives, 40 cars and trucks," the report noted. The Germans had still had plenty of firepower.

The scenes of liberation outside Veau's apartment window offered a joyous counter-narrative to 1940. He reported seeing a German car drive up rue de Miromesnil waving a white flag, and four Resistants marching past with a group of about fifty German soldiers, hands tied behind their necks. Just after noon, PVR and Milliez rode their bicycles to Paris City Hall to wait for General de Gaulle. In the early afternoon, General von Choltitz surrendered the Hotel Meurice; but Germans still held out at Hotel Majestic headquarters, and sporadic shooting was heard around the Luxembourg

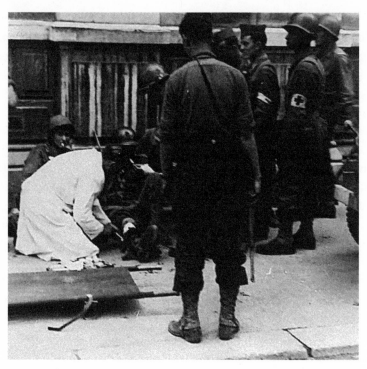

Doctors treating soldiers in Neuilly-sur-Seine during the liberation,
August 1944. Service Historique de la Défense.

Gardens. When de Gaulle finally arrived at City Hall around 6 p.m., the National Council of Resistance, along with PVR and Milliez, lined up to greet him. Council President Georges Bidault welcomed the general, calling him "the hope, the light and the surest guide" during the years of Occupation. De Gaulle responded with words that set the historical framework for the liberation for decades to come: "Paris! Paris humiliated! Paris broken! Paris martyred! But Paris liberated, liberated by herself, liberated by her people with the assistance of the armies of France, with the support and help of all of France, of France which fights, of the only France, of the true France, of the eternal France." Postwar politics meant seventy-five years would pass before the American role in the liberation was given its due at the new Musée de la Libération, opened on August 25, 2019, with a re-enactment of the Free French Second Armored Division's entry into the city. Rowdy *La Nueve* soldiers and elegant Rochambelles, the legendary women's ambulance unit, were represented among the division.

De Gaulle insisted in the immediate aftermath of the capital's liberation that the French Republic had not ceased to exist during the Occupation, that the Vichy government had been an aberration, and that he was now the President. With his iron will, intimidating stature, and deft undercutting of opposition, de Gaulle put a stop to the political squabbling. He led a parade of left, right, and center down the Champs-Elysées on August 26 to demonstrate who was in charge, both to the French people and to the US military leaders, who had refused General Leclerc permission to join the parade. De Gaulle was later quoted as saying he had loaned Leclerc to the Americans for the war and had simply borrowed him back for a few hours in Paris.

Amid the chaos of liberation, Elisabeth de La Bourdonnaye was trying to find her eldest son, Geoffroy, who had slipped out of France four years before to join the Free French. Now he was arriving in Paris with the Second Armored Division, and she couldn't wait to see him. He called her apartment the morning of August 25 and left word that he was coming into the city on rue Monge. Elisabeth flew. "He climbed down from his tank and to the amazement of the crowd on the sidewalk, he kissed me and then jumped back onto his tank and shouted '*Maman,* I have to go up rue Cujas and I don't remember where it is.' So I rode ahead of him on my bicycle," Elisabeth wrote in a postwar memoir.[13]

Elisabeth's daughter Bertranne d'Hespel, widowed at age nineteen in the fighting in 1939, now a medical student and key escape-line helper, jumped on her bicycle to join them. "I passed through whistling bullets, crossed over barricades, and finally arrived," she wrote in a memoir.[14] "I saw the tanks surrounding the Luxembourg, where the Germans had taken refuge, firing from time to time. I saw my mother, who pointed to an officer who advanced toward us. 'Don't you recognize your brother?' No, I did not recognize him. In 1940, he was a skinny adolescent with glasses who left for England. In 1944, I find an officer with broad shoulders."

That afternoon, with his regiment's tanks lined up in the Tuileries, Geoffroy introduced his sister and mother and Debré to his comrades. "Joy and pride to meet up with her son," Debré noted in his journal. "It was a happy moment." Bertranne wrote that she spent the day with her brother, catching up on all that happened in the intervening years, while keeping a wary eye on the Germans in the park. Geoffroy now was a lieutenant in the Free French Forces' 501st Regiment, commander of a tank squadron.

"At the end of the afternoon, the Germans raised a white flag over the

Senate and other places they were still occupying," Bertranne wrote. "Paris is free! Four years of occupation are over. The bells rang out the victory." Her work was not over, though. She was called in to hospital duty to help treat the scores of injuries from fighting that continued to erupt around the city. On September 8, Geoffroy and the rest of the Second Armored Division departed to finish what they started. German troops had abandoned Paris, but they still held eastern France.

Five months later, Elisabeth got word that Geoffroy had been badly wounded in an artillery attack at Grussenheim, in Alsace, on January 28, 1945. He died two days later, age twenty-three. Then in April 1945, as prisoners began returning from concentration camps, she learned that her son Guy, age nineteen, had died at Mauthausen in March, two months before its liberation. Elisabeth lost her two eldest sons at the end of the war, when she thought the worst was behind them. The joy of liberation was darkened by such devastating loss.

The morning after liberation, Dr. Veau awoke early and felt the difference in the air right away. "The street is not the same. They are no longer there. Other days at this time there were as many Germans in the street as French. You could hear their boots!"

The line in front of the bakery was still long, food was in short supply, and there was a mountain of work ahead to get Paris back on track, but the Nazis were gone. That was somewhere to start.

EPILOGUE

O n May 8, 1945, Germany signed its second surrender of the century. Peace had arrived, but Europe—in ruins physically, economically, and socially—was in poor condition to celebrate. Housing, food, heating fuel, and gasoline remained in short supply. Rationing tickets for buying bread, the most basic of French staples, remained in place through 1949. The Provisional Government ran the show until elections in October 1945 brought a leftist-dominated coalition to the National Assembly, provoking de Gaulle's resignation in January 1946. The Fourth Republic was off to a rocky start, but few had the stomach for a bitter political struggle. It was a time for healing and regrouping, and on so many levels, cleaning up the debris of four years of occupation.

As soon as Paris was liberated, revenge lashed out on a personal, extrajudicial level, and by the end of it an estimated ten thousand individuals paid the final price for their choices during the Occupation. Historians believe some assassinations were of a personal nature, using collaboration as a covering lie to be rid of an enemy, but how many? Impossible to know at this point. In the courts, another 310,000 French faced trials on charges ranging from plundering the property of others to "direct or indirect assistance to the Germans or their allies," the legal phrasing for the charge of collaboration. For cooperation with the enemy, a softer half-step away from collaboration, the charge was phrased as "damage to the national dignity." And for antisemitic acts, a long and appalling list, the charge was "damage to the unity of the French." Half the cases were dropped without further action. Some ten thousand French women had their heads shaved, some of them were marched naked through the streets, to punish what was referred to somewhat leeringly as "horizontal collaboration." About 20 percent of the national police force was fired.[1]

And the doctors? Most of the high-profile collaborators did not long survive. As mentioned previously, Alexis Carrel died of natural causes before he could be tried. Bernard Ménétrel, Pétain's highly influential personal physician, was among those who fled to Germany in the summer of 1944, of whom about two thousand wound up in Sigmaringen, where a vast Hohenzollern castle overlooking the Danube became the German-assigned home of Marshal Pétain. Upon his return to France in May 1945, Ménétrel spent six months in Fresnes prison before being released, and was eventually cleared by the court. He died of injuries sustained in a car accident in 1947.

Dr. Louis-Ferdinand Destouches, known as the writer Céline, worked as physician to the French refugees at Sigmaringen, along with Dr. André Jacquot, a right-wing militant from Remiremont in the Vosges region. Destouches then left Germany for Denmark, where he was arrested in December 1945, and spent eighteen months in prison and then three years on a work-release farm. In 1950, he was convicted in absentia in France of damage to the national dignity and sentenced to time served. He returned to France in 1951, wrote a book about his exile titled *D'un chateau l'autre* (*Castle to Castle*), and registered with the Medical Order to return to medical practice at his home in Meudon, a Paris suburb. He died in 1961.

George Montandon, the Gestapo's racial identity man, found gunmen at his door on August 3, 1944, before the city was liberated. They killed both him and his wife. Fernand Querrioux, rabidly antisemitic author of the "Medicine and the Jews" pamphlet, joined the rat pack at Sigmaringen and was killed nearby in an Allied bombing in April 1945.

With the Allies closing in on Sigmaringen, the Germans took Marshal Pétain and his entourage east and eventually handed him over to the Swiss. Escorted back to Paris by a French military contingent, he was imprisoned in the Fort de Montrouge. His trial, styled by one newspaper "The Greatest Trial in Our History," began July 23, 1945, in an overflowing Paris courtroom. Pétain was convicted of high treason and sentenced to death on August 15, 1945, but two days later de Gaulle commuted the sentence to life in prison, given Pétain's age. He lasted six years in fortress prisons off the Atlantic coast, slipping deeper and deeper into the dementia his friends claimed he had had since the start of the Occupation. He died in July 1951.

After Pétain's trial and conviction, the legal proceedings and extralegal revengefests tapered off. Forgive and forget was the new watchword for the French.

But in Nuremberg, the Nazi trials had just begun. On August 8, 1945, the United States, Great Britain, the USSR, and France formed an International Military Tribunal to try twenty-four Nazi leaders on charges in three categories: crimes against peace, war crimes, and crimes against humanity. Specific definitions of each were outlined in a formal agreement, and a procedure was agreed to by representatives of the four nations. Sentences handed down in October 1946 sent ten men to the hangman's noose, others to lengthy prison sentences. Those trials were followed in December 1946 by the so-called Doctors' Trial, in which twenty-two German men and one woman, twenty of them physicians, were accused of committing murder, torture, and atrocities on concentration camp prisoners. Among witnesses for the prosecution was Dr. Victor Dupont, who on January 28, 1946 (Day 44 of the trial), described in heart-wrenching detail the brutality of acts and conditions in Buchenwald. Death was a daily occurrence in the camp, but Dupont, the father of two children, said that watching a group of one hundred Tzigane (Roma) children being sent from Buchenwald to the gas chamber at Auschwitz remained his most tragic memory of his time there. "Those children knew perfectly well what awaited them, and they were shoved into the wagons while they screamed and cried."[2]

Dupont testified that at the time of his arrival in January 1944, the daily death toll was about a dozen, but as the numbers of incoming prisoners grew in winter 1945, those who could not work were sent to Block 61, where up to two hundred a day were put to death. Dr. Gerhard Schiedlausky and his assistants gave them a fatal injection of phenol acid in the heart. Their bodies were burned in the crematorium, and the ashes tossed in the latrine ditch, whose soil was then used for fertilizer in nearby fields.[3] Other subcamps had a system of hanging certain prisoners while obliging the rest of the camp to parade by their bodies. Dupont noted that in speaking with other liberated prisoners, he had learned of the consistency of killing methodology across the camp system. He believed that detailed orders for it were sent from the top Nazi leadership.

"In the precise case of Buchenwald, the personnel, however hard they could be, never had any initiative in their acts, and the *Lagerführer* [camp commander], the SS doctor himself, always took refuge behind their higher orders, often in a vague manner," Dupont said. "The name most frequently evoked was that of [SS Commander Heinrich] Himmler."[4]

The prosecutor asked specifically about interaction with German residents of the Weimar area around Buchenwald. Could they have known what went on at the camp? Dupont was precise: "Their ignorance, when the camps had existed for many years, was impossible." The prisoners were taken through public train stations, witnessed by other travelers. When they went to work details in outlying factories, they were put on duty with regular workers, who went home to their families at night. At Buchenwald, some German prisoners were allowed family visits. "It does not seem possible that the German population could deny having knowledge of the atrocities that occurred in the camps," Dupont said.[5] Yet many did.

In the Doctors' Trial, sixteen of the twenty physician defendants were found guilty, seven of them executed. The major result of the trial was the creation of the Nuremberg Code, which for the first time provided protocols for medical experimentation within humanitarian bounds, starting with informed consent. Going forward, no one could be the subject of a medical experiment without their consent, regardless of their judicial status.

Upon his return to Paris, Dupont went back to practicing medicine. He died in 1976. Charles Richet also went back to work, researching the effects of extended poor nutrition and damage done to deportees in the camps. In 1957 he published a monograph, *Pathologie de la Misère* (Pathology of Misery), on his findings. He died in 1966.

After the upheaval of surrender, occupation, and liberation, the path forward for France was uncertain. The Communist Party had gained momentum through its Resistance work, while the conservative right-wing parties had been undermined. The Gaullists tried to pull the weight toward the center, and to take advantage of the opportunity to bring about some badly needed reforms. In late 1944, between the liberation of Paris and the end of the war, Robert Debré put together proposals for changing the public health system and medical school education in France. He published them in a left-leaning newsletter called *Le Médecin français* (*The French Doctor*), which had begun as a clandestine publication by the National Front in 1941. In the October 25, 1944, issue he launched the idea that France needed a medical system "that will give each citizen, no matter their circumstances, the most advanced care."[6]

Just after the war, Debré was named council president for the National Institute of Hygiene (INH), a Vichy-created organization tasked with overseeing public health. At the time, hospitals and clinics had little research capability, as scientific exploration and clinical medicine were distinct fields. Debré insisted that medical research be brought into hospital work, as he did at Necker-Enfants Malades. One of his first acts at the INH was to hire as director biophysicist Louis Bugnard, a former Rockefeller Institute researcher, who immediately set up a grant program with the venerable New York center to host two French researchers a year. "It was in the United States, in particular, that our young researchers learned the techniques of utilization of radioisotopes in the laboratory and the hospital, new procedures such as electroencephalography (EEG) and neurophysiology, methods of exploring cardiovascular function, recent techniques in biochemistry," Bugnard said later.[7]

Under Vichy, the role of hospitals was shifted from nineteenth-century hospice for the poor to state-run health care open to all citizens, and in the immediate postwar period, health insurance for salaried workers, part of a larger social support package, was begun. But an extensive redesign of the medical system was put on hold. It would take eleven years before a group of young doctors, calling themselves the Friends of Radical Doctors association, picked up the ball. They began pushing for change, and when a new, forward-looking government was elected, they came knocking at Debré's door. Would he lead the reform effort? At seventy-four, retired from practicing, he was delighted to jump in, with certain conditions: he would not simply lead discussions, but would engage in action. Commission members would be chosen based on their competence in the subject, and not simply to represent a politically diverse front of unions and administrations. High-level government officials would be kept informed of decisions and recommendations. Debré noted that they were following a British model for effecting change, and he found it efficient and democratic, avoiding the public fuss that press campaigns or government-led initiatives for change often draw. It took them a little over a year. They rented office space in Saint Germain-des-Près and met weekly, holding round-table discussions and listening to experts. Discussions were at times heated, Debré wrote, as they included opponents of reform, whom he noted mostly were opposed to any change whatsoever.[8] The cornerstone of French conservatism is to maintain tradition and status quo, whether they work or not.

The first draft of the proposed reform, ready in July 1957, recommended turning public hospitals in towns with universities into teaching hospitals, soon named Centres Hospitaliers Universitaires (University Hospital Centers), known as CHUs. Medical students would no longer have to find a "mandarin"—an established doctor working in a private clinic and hospital—to take them on as residents before they could be certified for hospital practice. And doctors could work full-time at hospitals for a salary, rather than having to support unpaid hospital work through private practice. Charles de Gaulle signed the reform into law on December 30, 1958, two days before his extraordinary powers of ordinance would expire. A week later, France's Fifth Republic came into being, with de Gaulle as president and Robert's son Michel Debré as prime minister. Henceforth, laws and reforms would go through parliamentary process.

Had Robert Debré not been determined to reform the system, and had Michel Debré not been at the forefront of bringing about the new constitution, the change might never have happened, according to Jean Dausset, a member of the reform commission who went on to win the Nobel Prize in medicine in 1980. "It is likely that without the extraordinary coincidence of circumstances, that law would have had no chance of passing in the Chamber of Deputies, where the very powerful medical lobbies held sway," Dausset wrote later. "The son of Professor Debré applied himself to rapidly putting into operation his father's concepts, and he did it with great clarity and all efficiency, to which we owe a great deal."[9]

Today France counts thirty-two CHU hospital groups, including the extensive Paris-area network of thirty-nine hospitals. Health care is part of a vast social security system that ensures low-cost treatment for all, with government-controlled fees and prices, partly paid for through taxes on salaries. Multiple reforms have occurred since 1958, but maintaining a public health system has remained a priority for governments since.

Debré also was instrumental in getting UNICEF (United Nations International Childrens' Emergency Fund) off the ground, attending its organizational meeting in New York in 1946 as the French government representative, eager to help ease the misery of children in poverty around the world. He recounted being told by a Romanian representative that clothing and supplies were so sparse in his country that newborns in the midst of winter were wrapped in nothing more than a sheet of newspaper. The agency dispatched vitamins, medicine, clothing, and shoes for children to countries

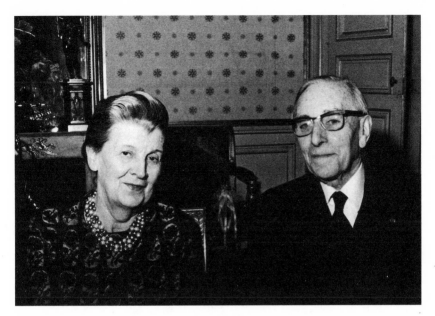

Robert Debré and Elisabeth de La Bourdonnaye, years after the war.
Collection of Geoffroy de Lassus.

across the globe. Once the postwar penury subsided, UNICEF moved on to distributing vaccines, especially for tuberculosis, and to augmenting nutrition for children in developing nations.[10]

Debré and Elisabeth de La Bourdonnaye were married in 1956 and saw their families grow and expand on both sides, with Robert counting eleven grandchildren and Elisabeth twenty-six, a half-dozen of whom became doctors. She died in 1972 and he followed in 1978.

After the war, Louis Pasteur Vallery-Radot went back to work at the Broussais Hospital in Paris and oversaw the founding of international branches of the Institut Pasteur. PVR was elected to the Académie Française, inducted in 1949. After he died in 1970, the Académie director offered a brief but poignant elegy: "He consecrated his life to the memory of his grandfather, who was his model; to the service of France, which was his passion; to music, which was his delight, and to friendship, which was his art."[11]

Paul Milliez, who remained PVR's assistant until he retired in 1959, went on to practice, teach, and lead various civic and medical organizations. He died in 1994. Robert Merle d'Aubigné founded a clinic dedicated to re-education and recovery from orthopedic surgery and also served on the boards of civic and medical organizations before his death in 1989. Alec Prochiantz became chief of pediatric surgery at the American Hospital of Paris and pioneered various surgical techniques that bear his name. He joined the Air Force Escape and Evasion Society (AFEES) and attended reunions in the United States with veterans he had helped to safety during the war. He died in 2013 at the age of 99.

For all the doctors of the Resistance, their work during the Occupation remained a highlight of their lives, a moment when their nation, their families, and their own integrity had called them to act, and they had found the courage and resilience to do so. They had not lacked in leadership before the war, but they were confirmed in it afterward. Grateful communities across the country honored them by giving their names to streets, squares, hospitals, and clinics; they were decorated with the highest medals and citations. They continued to look forward and to work for a better world. PVR, in his 1949 speech to the Académie Française, reminded its august members that the victory of France, through its darkest night, with the aid of its allies, would remain a beacon of promise to others:

"May the France of today, steeped in a past of 20 centuries, proud of the fight that it sustained to recover its liberty, and loyal to the spirit of Charles de Gaulle, provide for humanity in distress a new ideal, a reason to live, and to hope."[12]

NOTES

INTRODUCTION

1. Jean-Paul Sartre, "The Truth about Occupied Paris," *Tricolor Magazine* (January 1945).

2. The "Loi portant statut de juifs" (Law establishing the status of Jews), dated October 3, 1940, became law when it was published in the *Journal Officiel* on October 18, 1940. It defined who would be considered Jewish, and listed public-service positions from which they were henceforth barred, with a narrow exception for military service.

3. Pierre Lefebvre, "Le Service de santé militaire à la veille de la Campagne de France en 1940," conference given March 1990 to the Société française d'Histoire de la Médecine, https://www.biusante.parisdescartes.fr/sfhm/hsm/HSMx1990x024x003_4/HSMx1990x024 x003_4x0173.pdf.

4. Anne Simonin, "Le Comité Médicale de la Résistance," in *La Résistance, une histoire sociale,* ed. Antoine Prost (Paris: Editions de l'Atélier, 1997), 166.

5. Letter from George Montandon, April 26, 1940, Centre de Documentation Juive Contemporaine (CDJC) XCV-114.

6. Serge Klarsfeld, *Mémorial de la Déportation des Juifs de France* (Paris: Fondation Fils et Filles de Déportés Juifs de France, 2012), foreword.

7. Isabelle von Bueltzingsloewen, "Rationing and Politics: The French Academy of Medicine and Food Shortages during the German Occupation and the Vichy Regime," in *Food and War in Twentieth-Century Europe* (Surrey, England: Ashgate Publishing Ltd. 2011), 165.

1. THE SHOCKING COLLAPSE

1. Pierre Lefebvre, "Le Service de santé militaire à la veille de la Campagne de France en 1940," conference given March 1990 to the Société française d'Histoire de la Médecine, https://www.biusante.parisdescartes.fr/sfhm/hsm/HSMx1990x024x003_4/HSMx1990x024 x003_4x0173.pdf.

2. Lefebvre, "Le Service de santé militaire."

3. See Fabrice Virgili, "Peurs, déréglements et désordres, le 14 juin 1940 à l'hôpital d'Orsay," in *L'Historien et les relations internationales, Autour de Robert Frank* (Publications de la Sorbonne, 2012).

4. Bullitt to FDR, June 12, 1940, FDR Library and Museum, http://docs.fdrlibrary.marist. edu/psf/box2/t12am01.html.

5. Robert Murphy, *Diplomat among Warriors* (New York: Doubleday, 1964), 45.

6. William C. Bullitt Papers, MS 112, Box 22, Series 1, Yale University Library.

7. Paul Richey, *Fighter Pilot. A Personal Record of the Campaign in France 1939–1940* (The History Press [reprint], 2016). Kindle.

8. *Foreign Relations of the United States,* telegram from Bullitt to the Secretary of State, July 1, 1940, https://history.state.gov/historicaldocuments/frus1940v02/d536.

9. Henri Nahum, *La Médecine française et les Juifs 1930–1945* (Paris: Editions L'Harmattan, 2006), 170.

10. Nicolas Chevassus-au-Louis, *Savants sous l'Occupation* (Paris: Perrin, 2004), 97–98.

11. Robert Vial, *Histoire des Hôpitaux de Paris sous l'Occupation* (Paris: L'Harmattan, 1999), 30.

12. Nahum, *La Médecin française,* 153.

13. Dr. Raymond Armbruster, a senator, introduced the measure to require doctors to pass the French high-school *baccalauréat* exam and graduate from a French medical school. Candidates would have to be born in France, or to have been naturalized French for five years before beginning studies, or to have fought for France in WWI. Aimed largely at Romanian immigrants, the law imposed a cap of ten Romanian medical students per year. In 1935, the Cousin-Nast law blocked naturalized doctors from practicing in the Public Assistance system for five years and required a four-year waiting period for those with no military service (such as women). For more detail, see Julie Fette, *Exclusions. Practicing Prejudice in French Law and Medicine 1920–45* (Ithaca, NY: Cornell University Press, 2012).

14. Von Bueltzingsloewen, "Rationing and Politics," 155.

15. Jean-Paul Sartre, *The Truth about Occupied Paris,* 1945.

16. Thomas Fontaine and Denis Peschanski, *La Collaboration. Vichy, Paris, Berlin, 1940–1945* (Paris: Tallandier-Archives Nationales-Ministère de la Défense, 2014).

2. THE RACIALIZATION OF HATRED

1. Vicky Caron, *Uneasy Asylum: France and the Jewish Refugee Crisis, 1933–1942* (Stanford, CA: Stanford University Press, 1999), 213.

2. Renée Poznanski, *Les Juifs en France pendant la Seconde Guerre mondiale* (Paris: Hachette, 1994; CNRS édition 2018), 30.

3. Nahum, *La Médecine française,* 86.

4. The Marchandeau Law, adopted in April 1939 at the request of the International League against Racism and Anti-Semitism, allowed prosecution of the press for "defamation or insult committed against a group of persons belonging, by their origins, to a specified race or religion, with the goal of arousing hatred between citizens or inhabitants (Lorsque la diffamation ou l'injure, commise envers un groupe de personnes appartenant, par leur origine, à une race ou à une religion déterminée, aura eu pour but d'exciter à la haine entre les citoyens ou les habitants)." The Vichy government repealed it on August 27, 1940.

5. *Au Pilori,* August 19, 1940.

6. Robert Debré journal 1940–1941, unpublished, Patrice Debré Archives.

7. Patrice Debré, *Robert Debré. Une vocation française* (Paris: Odile Jacob, 2018), 37–45.

8. Robert Debré, *L'Honneur de vivre* (Paris: Hermann, Editeurs des Sciences et des Arts, 1996), 222.

9. Archives nationales (AN) 13W/290.33.

10. Robert Debré, private journal, December 22, 1940.

11. *Bulletin de l'Ordre des Médecins 1941–1944* (Paris: Masson, 1941–2008), 129.

12. AN 13W/290.33/122–125.

13. Bruno Halioua, "La xénophobie et l'antisémitisme dans le milieu médical sous l'Occupation vus au travers du Concours Médical," Médecine/Sciences, Paris, 19(1) (January 2003): 107–115.

14. *Bulletin de l'Ordre des Médecins,* 130.

15. *Le Médecin français,* No. 12, April 1942.

16. AN AJ 40 555 (VKULT 401).

17. Jérôme Carcopino, *Souvenirs de sept ans* (Paris: Flammarion, 1953), 360.

18. Louis Halphen, historian; Jules Bloch, professor of linguistics; and Max Aron, doctor-researcher, went into hiding in the south and survived. Marc Bloch, historian and professor, and Paul Reiss, doctor-researcher, joined the Resistance, were caught by Germans and executed. André Mayer, doctor, and René Wurmser, biologist, escaped to the United States. Marc Klein, medical doctor-researcher, was deported to Auschwitz and survived. Paul Job, chemist, sent to Drancy in August 1944, also survived.

19. Debré, *L'Honneur de vivre,* 221.

20. CDJC CCXIX-104.

21. Nahum, *La Médecine française,* 101.

22. *La Presse Médicale,* No. 30, June 29, 1946. Obituary notice written by Pierre Hillemand.

23. CDJC XIe-51.

3. DANGER TAKES SHAPE

1. Louis Pasteur Vallery-Radot, *Mémoires d'un non-conformist* (Paris: Plon, 1966), 257.

2. Pasteur Vallery-Radot, Mémoires, 269.

3. Pasteur Vallery-Radot, introduction to Mémoires.

4. *Au Pilori,* September 13, 1940.

5. Debré, *L'Honneur de vivre,* 47.

6. Debré, *L'Honneur de vivre,* 223.

7. Yvonne Oddon, "Rapport sur mon activité," in *Sur les Camps de Déportées* (Paris: Editions Allia, 2021), 59.

8. Charles de Gaulle, June 18, 1940, speech: "Quoi qu'il arrive, la flamme de la résistance française ne doit pas s'éteindre et ne s'éteindra pas."

9. The full quote from Napoléon Bonaparte was: "La mort n'est rien, mais vivre dans la défaite et sans gloire c'est mourir quotidiennement." Several Resistance newsletters and publications borrowed the shorter version as a slogan.

10. Paul Milliez, *Médecin de la Liberté* (Paris: Editions du Seuil, 1982), 43.

11. Debré, private journal, March 23, 1941.

12. Debré, private journal, March 25, 1941.

13. Lorraine Colin, *De châteaux en prison, la vie d'Elisabeth de La Panouse-Debré* (Paris: L'Harmattan, 2021), 138.

14. Colin, *De châteaux en prison,* 152. "Entourée héroïnes otages, condamnées à mort; moral merveilleux."

15. Debré, *L'Honneur de vivre,* 226.

16. Robert Merle d'Aubigné, *Une Trace* (Paris: La Table Ronde, 1987), 141.

17. Merle d'Aubigné, *Une Trace,* 142.

18. Rose and Philippe d'Estienne d'Orves, *Honoré d'Estienne d'Orves: Pionnier de la Résistance. Papiers, carnets et lettres* (Paris: Editions France-Empire, 1985), annex.

19. Debré, private journal, December 13, 1940.

20. Debré, *L'Honneur de vivre,* 222.

21. Debré, *L'Honneur de vivre,* 239.

22. Debré, *L'Honneur de vivre,* 228.

23. Christian Chevandier, *Infirmières parisiennes 1900–1950: Emergence d'une profession* (Paris: Publications de la Sorbonne, 2016), chap. 6.

24. CDJC CXVI-65.

25. CDJC XXIII-12.

26. Debré, *L'Honneur de vivre,* 240.

27. André Chaumet, "Demain au Palais Berlitz s'ouvre l'exposition 'La France et le Juif,'" *Paris Soir,* September 5, 1941, 1. "Elle ne fait preuve d'aucune passion, d'aucun ressentiment, d'aucune haine. Elle se contente de montrer purement et simplement, sans commentaires, la position des juifs en France, leurs main-mise profonde sur tous les leviers de commande de l'activité politique, littéraire et économique de la France."

28. *Le Médecin français,* No. 1, March 1941, "Pourquoi ce journal?" 1. "Nous lutterons de toutes nos forces contre toutes les formes d'obscurantisme et toutes les formes d'étouffement de la pensée, d'où qu'elles viennent. Nous lutterons pour que notre pays aux si riches traditions reprenne la tête du progrès. Nous lutterons contre l'oppression nationale, pour la liberté et l'indépendance de la France."

29. *Le Médecin français,* No. 1, March 1941, "Les Hommes de la Révolution Nationale: No. 1—Querrioux Fernand," 2. "M. Querrioux est un médecin malhonnête, un politicien taré, et il est assez caractéristique qu'il soit l'homme de la 'Revolution National.'"

30. Fernand Querrioux, "Triomphe du Juif ou Périr," *Le Matin,* September 15, 1941, 1. "Le médecin pénètre dans l'existence familiale, dans les secrets des foyers, dans l'intimité des personnes; au cours d'une carrière qui est, le plus souvent, un véritable apostolat, le médecin reçoit les confidences les plus délicates, il lui faut souvent soigner le moral, en même temps que le corps, de ses malades."

4. RESISTANCE SPREADS ROOTS

1. Dupont wrote detailed postwar reports on the Vengeance network, kept in the archives of the Service Historique de la Défense at Vincennes. He also gave several interviews about his work, available online on the resourceful website of historian Marc Chantran, http://chantran.vengeance.free.fr/Doc/VicDupontv14.pdf.

2. Admiral Leahy to State Department, November 19, 1941, https://history.state.gov/historicaldocuments/frus1941v02/d397.

3. Merle d'Aubigné, *Une Trace,* 146.

4. Merle d'Aubigné, *Une Trace,* 145.

5. Merle d'Aubigné, *Une Trace,* 146.

6. The oath is a formula still in legal use in France today for various attestations, including recently the need to go outside during confinement for the COVID-19 pandemic.

7. Merle d'Aubigné, *Une Trace,* 138.

8. Marc Knobel, "George Montandon et l'ethno-racisme," in *L'anti-sémitism de plume,* 279.

9. Henri Nahum, *La Médecine française,* 147.

10. Merle d'Aubigné, *Une Trace,* 139.

11. Milliez, *Médecin de la Liberté,* 46.

12. CDJC CCXXXVIII-117.

13. Renée Poznanski, *Les Juifs en France pendant la Seconde Guerre Mondiale* (Paris: CNRS Editions, 2018), 365.

14. CDJC CCXXXVIII-117.

15. CDJC XXIII-17b.

16. Calculating the equivalence of the Occupation-era French franc to the value of today's dollar is fairly meaningless. The Germans installed an official exchange of 20 FF to 1 Reichsmark; in 1944 the exchange rate on the black market was 288 FF to $1; after liberation the official rate was set at 50 FF to $1. The value of goods varied widely, depending on whether they were bought on the official market with ration tickets, from a friend, or on the black market. For more detail on the Occupation economy, see Louis Baudin, *Esquisse sur l'économie française sous l'occupation allemande* (Paris: Editions Politiques, Economique et Sociales, Librairie de Médicis, 1945).

17. François Wetterwald, *Vengeance: Histoire d'un corps franc* (Paris: Mouvement Vengeance, 1946), 48. A version of the book is also available online: http://chantran.vengeance.free.fr/Doc/Wetterwaldv50.pdf.

18. AN F/1a/3859–3860 BCRA Santé Publique.

19. AN F/1a/3760 Service de Santé.

20. Wetterwald, *Histoire d'un corps-franc,* 61–63.

21. Wetterwald, *Histoire d'un corps-franc,* 32.

22. Victor Dupont interviews, http://chantran.vengeance.free.fr/Doc/VicDupontv14.pdf, 20.

23. La Contemporaine F/delta/res/0844/11.

24. Prochiantz interview with Sylvie Zaidman and Joseph Clesse, Archives de Seine-Saint Denis, 1994, audio, 1AV/2399.

25. Prochiantz interview.

26. Prochiantz interview.

27. James E. Armstrong, *Escape!* (Spartanburg, SC: Honoribus Press, 2000), 59–60.

28. Armstrong, *Escape!* 212.

29. Prochiantz interview.

30. Prochiantz interview.

31. Merle d'Aubigné, *Une Trace,* 148–49.

32. Pierre Canlorbe, *La Service de Santé de la Résistance* (Paris: PhD diss., Ecole de Médecine de Paris, 1945).

33. Milliez, *Médecin de la Liberté,* 43.

1. Von Bueltzingsloewen, "Rationing and Politics," 162.

2. Heinz Hohenwald, Guy Krivopissko, and Daniel Virieux, *La Résistance. La Liberté en Héritage* (Paris: Messidor/La Farandole, Conseil Général du Val-de-Marne, 1990), 72.

3. Von Bueltzingsloewen, "Rationing and Politics," 165.

4. *Bulletin de l'Ordre des Médecins,* Volume 1941–44, 59.

5. *Bulletin,* 163.

6. Charles Richet, *Trois Bagnes* (Paris: J. Ferenczi et fils, 1945), introduction.

7. AN 72 AJ F/1a/3859–3860.

8. AN 72 AJ F/1a/3859–3860.

9. AN 72 AJ F/1a/3859–3860.

10. AN 72 AJ F/1a/3760.

11. AN 72 AJ F/1a/3760.

12. AN 72 AJ F/1a/3760.

13. AN 72 AJ F/1a/3760.

14. AN 72 AJ F/1a/3721.

15. AN 72 AJ F/1a/3721.

16. CJDC CCXXXIII-646.

17. CJDC CCXXXIII-646.

18. CJDC CCXXXIII-646.

19. Nahum, *La Médecine française et les Juifs,* 288.

20. Charles-Jean Odic, *'Stepchildren' of France* (New York: Roy Publishers, 1945), 101.

21. Debré, *L'Honneur de vivre,* 232.

22. Colette Brull-Ulmann, *Les Enfants de la Dernier Salut* (Paris: City Editions, 2017), Kindle, Chapter 10.

23. Brull-Ulmann, *Les Enfants,* chap. 15.

24. Brull-Ulmann, *Les Enfants,* chap. 14.

25. Odic, *'Stepchildren,'* 55.

26. Brull-Ulmann, *Les Enfants,* chap. 11.

27. CJDC CCXXXIII-49.

28. CJDC CCXXXIII-646.

29. While Katharine Meyer Graham wrote in a memoir that Bertrand Zadoc-Kahn was chief medical officer at The American Hospital of Paris, the hospital has no record of him. He may have consulted there on occasion.

6. PERSECUTION INTENSIFIES

1. Report of Dr. Jean Tisné, 7 September 1941, CDJC CII-8.

2. Tisné, CDJC CII-8.

3. Report of Dr. Jean Tisné, February 10, 1942, AN F/7/15107.

4. Tisné, AN F/7/15107.

5. Report of Dr. Samuel Steinberg, AN F/9/5577. The SRCGE (Enemy War Crimes Research Service) was created in October 1944 and interviewed hundreds of victims of and witnesses to Nazi terror. It was disbanded in 1948.

6. Charles Odic, *'Stepchildren,'* 164.

7. CDJC CCXVI-66.

8. CDJC CCXVI-66.

9. CDJC CCXVI-66.

10. For more detail on the Vittel camp, see the *Anonymes, Justes et Persécutés durant la période Nazie* website, http://www.ajpn.org/internement-camp-de-vittel-215.html.

11. Jean-Jacques Bernard, *Le Camp de la mort lente: Compiègne 1941–1942* (Paris: Editions Le Manuscrit, 2006), 156.

12. Bernard, *Le Camp,* 158.

13. *La Lettre Sépharade,* No. 35, http://www.lalettresepharade.fr/home/la-revue-par-num ero/numero-35/simon-lubicz.

14. "Rescue of Jews: One and All," Yad Vashem exhibits website, https://www.yadvashem .org/yv/en/exhibitions/rescue-by-jews/lubicz.asp.

15. See the US Holocaust Memorial and Museum website for more information on Auschwitz, https://encyclopedia.ushmm.org/content/en/article/auschwitz.

16. André Charles Marsault notice, Amis de La Fondation de la Résistance website, https:// www.memoresist.org/resistant/andre-charles-marsault/.

17. Edmond Michelet, *Rue de la Liberté. Dachau 1943–45* (Genève: Editions de Crémille, 1971), 254.

18. Michelet, *Rue de la Liberté,* 255.

19. Adélaïde Hautval dossier, La Contemporaine, F/delta/res/797/53.

20. Adélaïde Hautval, *Médecine et Crimes Contre l'Humanité* (Paris: Actes Sud, 1991), 78.

21. Adélaïde Hautval entry, Encylopedia.com, https://www.encyclopedia.com/women/ency clopedias-almanacs-transcripts-and-maps/hautval-adelaide-1906-1988.

22. Hautval entry, Encyclopedia.com.

7. PRISONERS OF HATRED

1. See the US Holocaust Memorial Museum website for more information on the concentration camp system. The figure of more than forty thousand camps includes internment, prisoner-of-war, and concentration camps, some of which were set up in 1933 and later dismantled. After 1942, the larger concentration camps also counted a system of subcamps under their administration. For example, Buchenwald had more than 130 subcamps organized for slave labor by 1945. https://encyclopedia.ushmm.org/content/en/article/concentration-camp -system-in-depth.

2. The exact number of doctors who were deported to Buchenwald or any other camp is not known; historians estimate that between 300 and 500 doctors overall were deported during the war.

3. Jean Rousset, *Chez les barbares* (Lyon: Editions de la Guillotière, 1946), 14.

4. Dominique Orlowski, dir., *Buchenwald Par Ses Témoins* (Paris: Belin, 2014), 436.

5. Orlowski, *Buchenwald,* 382.

6. Christian Bernadac, *Médecins de l'impossible* (Editions France-Empire, 1967), 294.

7. Rousset, *Chez les barbares,* 15.

8. Richet, *Trois Bagnes,* 50.

9. Charles-Jean Odic, *Demain Buchenwald* (Paris: Buchet-Chastel, 1972), 17–19.

10. Olga Wormser and Henri Michel, *Tragédies de la Déportation 1940–45. Témoignages des survivants des camps de concentration allemands* (Paris: Hachette, 1955), 300, footnote.

11. Frédéric-Henri Manhès, *Buchenwald: L'Organisation et L'Action Clandestine des Déportés Français 1944–1945* (Paris: FNDIRP (Fédération nationale des déportés et internés, résistants et patriotes), 1947), 15.

12. Olivier Lalieu, *La Zone Grise? La Résistance française à Buchenwald* (Paris: La Grande Livre du mois), 148.

13. Lucien Cariat, *Ici, chacun son dû* (Paris: La Pensée universelle, 1973), 66–67.

14. Victor Dupont, "Réflexions sur le Sens des Camps de Concentrations Nazis," in Robert Antelme, *Les Vivants* (Paris: Boivin, 1945), 48.

15. Dupont, "Réflexions," 44.

16. Dupont, "Réflexions," 55–56.

17. *Procès des Grands Criminels de Guerre devant le Tribunal Militaire International à Nuremberg* (14 novembre 1945–1 octobre 1946, Tome VI), 267.

18. Charles Richet, *Trois Bagnes,* 65.

19. Richet, *Trois Bagnes,* 58.

20. Richet, *Trois Bagnes,* 47.

21. Pierre Bretonneau, *Témoignage,* Association Française Buchenwald-Dora et Kommandos website, https://asso-buchenwald-dora.com/temoignage-de-pierre-bretonneau/.

22. Orlowski, *Buchenwald,* 157.

23. Manhès, *Buchenwald,* 47–48.

24. Report of Marcel Renet, AN F/9/5577.

25. Manhès, *Buchenwald,* 49.

26. Manhès, *Buchenwald,* 54–55.

27. Report of Michel Léon-Kindberg, AN F/9/5577. He was interviewed on May 2, 1945, and died six days later.

28. Blog, Coordination Liberté Egalité Fraternité (CLEF), https://laclef.typepad.fr/coordi nation_libert_galit/toussaint-gallet.html.

8. BLOOD IN THE FOREST

1. Alec Prochiantz, *Promenons-nous dans les bois* (Paris: Société des écrivains, 2011), 31–37.

2. Operation Houndsworth summary reports, http://ww2talk.com/index.php?threads/re port-operation-houndsworth.35231/.

3. Prochiantz, *Promenons-nous,* 107.

4. Ian Wellsted, *SAS with the Maquis: In Action with the French Resistance* (London: Frontline Books, 2016), 62.

5. Prochiantz, *Promenons-nous,* 51.

6. Marcel Vigreux, *Les villages-martyrs de Bourgogne: 1944* (Saulieu: Association pour la recherche sur l'Occupation et la Résistance, 1994), 81–82.

7. Wellsted, *SAS with the Maquis,* 87.

8. René Marin, *Un Enfant a vécu le massacre de Dun-les-Places (Juin 1944): Il raconte* (Self-published, 2015), 14.

9. Prochiantz interview, Archives de Seine-Saint-Denis, 1AV/2399.

10. Anita Winter letter, website of the Fondation de la Résistance, Musée de la Résistance en ligne, http://museedelaresistanceenligne.org/musee/doc/pdf/231.pdf.

11. Prochiantz, *Promenons-nous,* 75.

12. Prochiantz, *Promenons-nous,* 93.

13. Prochiantz, *Promenons-nous,* 97.

14. The film clip is visible here: https://www.youtube.com/watch?time_continue=122&v=GE-fQRhhumU.

15. Jacques Canaud, *Le Temps des Maquis* (Paris: De Borée, 2011), 161.

16. Wellsted, *SAS with the Maquis,* 107.

17. Wellsted, *SAS with the Maquis,* 108.

18. Joël Drogland, *Des Maquis du Morvan au Piège de la Gestapo: André Rondenay, Agent de la France Libre,* (Paris: Vendémiaire, 2019), 96.

19. Wellsted, *SAS with the Maquis,* 89.

20. Canaud, *Le Temps des Maquis,* 161.

21. Wellsted, *SAS with the Maquis,* 93.

22. Prochiantz, *Promenons-nous,* 88.

23. Wellsted, *SAS with the Maquis,* 157–58.

24. Hubert Cloix, *Les Maquis de Morvan,* http://mvr.asso.fr/front_office/fiche.php?idFiche=793&TypeFiche=4.

25. Cloix, *Les Maquis de Morvan.*

26. Prochiantz, *Promenons-nous,* 31–33.

27. Prochiantz, *Promenons-nous,* 34.

28. Claude Monod, *La Région D. Rapport d'activité des Maquis de Bourgogne-Franche-Comté (mai–septembre 1944)* (Saint-Etienne-Vallée-Française: Aiou, 1993), 46.

29. Monod, *La Région D,* 80.

30. Monod, *La Région D,* 108.

9. AN AMERICAN DOCTOR PITCHES IN

1. Clémence Bock, "Recollections of Dr. Jackson," Jackson Family Archives, 1.

2. A documentary film directed by Antony Easton, "The American in Paris," recounts the hospital's WWI service. It is available for viewing at: https://www.american-hospital.org/en/page/american-hospital-paris-during-great-war.

3. Bock, "Recollections," 3, 10.

4. Chambrun report to the American Hospital board of directors, December 1944, Archives of the American Hospital of Paris.

5. Film *Le Dossier du Doctor Jackson,* by Richard Lerchbaum and Ricardo Vega (2015), https://www.youtube.com/watch?v=eZeODPqJiQQ&feature=youtu.be.

6. Joseph Manos report, National Archives and Records Administration, College Park, Md., Escape and Evasion Reports Series No. 234.

7. Joseph Manos report.

8. Dossier Gilbert Asselin, SHD GR 16 P 19616.

9. Film *Le Dossier du Doctor Jackson.*

10. Bock, "Recollections," 14.

11. Charles-Julien Kaufmann, *L'Entreprise de la Mort Lente* (PhD diss., Ecole de Médecine de Nancy, Nancy: Imprimérie Nanciénne, 1946).

12. Folke Bernadotte, *The Curtain Falls: Last Days of the Third Reich* (New York: Alfred A. Knopf, 1945), 81.

13. George Martelli, *The Man Who Saved London* (New York: Doubleday, 1961), 246.

14. Report dated May 8, 1945, by Phillip Jackson, Jackson Family Archives.

15. SHD GR 16 P 34823.

16. AN/40/757.

17. Reports of the 365th Station Hospital, February to December 1945, US Army Office of Medical History.

10. LIBERATION AT LAST

1. Victor Veau Diary, MS 794 (1665), Bibliothèque de l'Académie Nationale de Médecine.

2. AN F/1a/3760.

3. Annette Monod interview, 1995, "Libération du camp de Drancy," https://www.ina.fr/video/P19207480.

4. Robert Monod, *Les Heures Décisives de la Libération de Paris (9–26 Août 1944)* (Paris: Editions Gilbert, 1947), 61.

5. Robert Debré, *L'Honneur de vivre,* 252.

6. Monod, *Les Heures Décisives,* 47.

7. AN F/1a/3760.

8. Milliez, *Médecin de la liberté,* 71–72.

9. Dietrich von Choltitz, *De Sébastopol à Paris: Un soldat parmi les soldats* (Paris: Aubanel, 1964), 244.

10. Roger Cocteau-Gallois, interview, http://museedelaresistanceenligne.org/media6029-A-propos-de-la-Lib.

11. Monod, *Les Heures Décisives,* 70.

12. A. de Chambrun, report to the board of The American Hospital of Paris, Hospital archives.

13. Geoffroy de Lassus, *Deux frères, un même engagement,* https://drive.google.com/file/d/1mcmdRQSpekJ0hKoMcjdptAUP746AIRYU/view.

14. Bertranne d'Hespel Auvert, Memoir, MS 1144(2015), Bibliothèque de l'Académie Nationale de Médecine.

EPILOGUE

1. François Rouquet et Fabrice Virgili, *Les Françaises, les Français et l'Épuration: de 1940 à nos jours* (Paris: Gallimard, 2018), 136, 150–51.

2. *Procès des Grand Criminels de Guerre devant le Tribunal Militaire International* (Nuremberg: Tribunal Militaire International, 1946–49, Vol. VI), 253.

3. *Procès des Grand Criminels,* 254–57.

4. *Procès des Grand Criminels,* 261.

5. *Procès des Grand Criminels,* 262.

6. Gérard Milhaud, "Les Conditions de réussite d'une grande réforme: la création des centres hospito-universitaires en 1958," *La Revue Administrative,* no. 354, Nov. 2006.

7. Institute Nationale de Santé et Recherche Médicale (INSERM) history page, https://histoire.inserm.fr/de-l-inh-a-l-inserm/l-institut-national-d-hygiene/les-annees-1945-1964.

8. Robert Debré, *L'Honneur de vivre,* 349.

9. Jean Dausset, Comments on the 50th anniversary of the creation of CHUs, https://francearchives.fr/commemo/recueil-2008/40067.

10. Robert Debré, *L'Honneur de vivre,* 329.

11. Maurice Druon, *Discours,* 15 octobre 1970, to the Académie Française.

12. Louis Pasteur Vallery-Radot, *Discours,* 28 mai 1946, to the Académie Française.

BIBLIOGRAPHY

PRIMARY SOURCES

Among the many archives consulted, the following were most pertinent.

Archives Nationales de France, Pierrefitte (AN)

    Exemptions made for Robert Debré and nine other prominent Jewish professors, AJ 40 555 (VKULT 401)

    Dossiers on the BRCA, Service de Santé de la Résistance, Maquis, AJ 72/F/1a/3859–3860, 3720–21, 3729, 3760

    Report of Dr. Jean Tisné, 10 February 1942, F/7/15107

    Report of Michel Léon-Kindberg, 2 May 1945, F/9/5577

    German documents from during the Occupation, AJ 40/757, 555, 885, 897, 899

    Documents from the WWII Historical Committee, AJ 72/35, 71

    Reports from doctors deported to concentration camps, F/9/5565–5577

    Correspondence between René Leriche and Bernard Ménétrel, 1940, 3W/289–293

Archives de La Contemporaine, Nanterre

    Fonds Charles Richet, BDIC-Arch 0059

    Fonds Turma-Vengeance, F/delta/res/0844/1–16

    Dossier Adélaïde Hautval, F/delta/res/797/53

Archives of the Service Historique de la Défense, Vincennes and Caen (SHD)

    Dossier Victor Dupont, G 16 P 202042

    Dossiers Sumner Jackson, GR 16 P 34823, AC 21 P 464681

    Dossier Robert Merle D'Aubigné, G 16 P 412667

    Dossier Paul Milliez, GR 16 P 419798

    Dossier Charles Richet, GR 16 P 510249

    Dossier François Wetterwald, G 16 P 295761

    Dossier Gilbert Asselin, GR 16 P 19616

    Dossier *Goélette* network, GR 17 P 136

Contemporary Jewish Documentation Center, Mémorial de la Shoah, Paris (CDJC)

    Letter from George Montandon, 26 April 1940, XCV-114

    Letter from Robert Debré and other Jewish WWI veterans to Pétain,
        CCXIX-104

    Letter from André Cachera requesting exclusion of Raymond Leibovici,
        CXVI-65

    Reports, letters and other material concerning Jewish doctors, XXIII-9–29

    Police report on Robert Debré not wearing yellow star, CCXXXVIII-117

    Reports by doctors and administration, Rothschild Hospital, CCXXXIII-646,
        49, 654, 48

    Report by Dr. Jean Tisné, 7 September 1941, CII-8

    Report by Dr. Abraham Drucker, 1946, CCXVI-66

Archives of the Bibliothèque de l'Académie Nationale de Médecine, Paris

    Diary of Victor Veau, MS 794 (1665)

    Journal of Bertranne Auvert, MS 1144 (2015)

    Biographical dossiers

Archives of The American Hospital of Paris, Neuilly-sur-Seine

    Board of governors reports, 1939–1941

    History of The American Hospital of Paris by Otto Gresser

Archives of Mémorial de l'internement et de la déportation, Camp de Royallieu,
    Compiègne

Yale University Archives, William Bullitt Papers, MS 112

Journal, 1940–1942, Robert Debré, from the archives of Patrice Debré

Oral interview with Alec Prochiantz, by Sylvie Zaidman and Joel Clesse, Archives de
    Seine-Saint-Denis, 1AV/2399

Sumner Jackson Family Archives

    Clémence Bock, "Recollections of Dr. Jackson"

Interviews with Patrice Debré, Marianne Debré, Lorraine Colin, Florence Prochiantz,
    Dominique Durand, René Marin, Noëlle Renault

Newspapers from 1940 to 1945, including *Au Pilori, Paris Soir, Le Matin, Le Combat
    Médical, Le Médecin français,* and *l'Ethnie française,* at the Bibliothèque Nationale
    de France

SECONDARY SOURCES

Antelme, Robert. *Les Vivants.* Paris: Boivin, 1945.

Baudin, Louis. *Esquisse sur l'économie française sous l'occupation allemande.* Paris: Editions Politiques, Economique, et Sociales, Librairie de Médicis, 1945.

Bernard, Jean-Jacques. *Le camp de la mort lente.* Paris: L'Edition Manuscrit, 2006.

Bernadec, Christian. *Les médecins de l'impossible.* Paris: Editions France-Empire, 1967.

Brull-Ulmann, Colette. *Les Enfants du Dernier Salut.* Paris: City Editions, 2017.

Bulletin de l'Ordre des Médecins 1941–1944. Paris: Masson, 1941–2008.

Canlorbe, Pierre. *La Service Santé de la Résistance,* PhD diss., Ecole de Médecine, 1945.

Cariat, Lucie. *Ici, chacun son dû.* Paris: La pensée universelle, 1973.

Caron, Vicki. *Uneasy Asylum: France and the Jewish Refugee Crisis 1993–42.* Stanford, CA: Stanford University Press, 1999.

Choltitz, Dietrich von. *De Sébastopol à Paris. Un soldat parmi les soldats.* Paris: Aubanel, 1964. Translated from the German by A.-M. Bécourt, Martin Briem, Klaus Diel and Pierre Michel.

Colin, Lorraine. *De Châteaux en prison, la vie d'Elisabeth de La Panouse-Debré.* Paris: L'Harmattan, 2021.

Debré, Patrice. *Robert Debré: Une vocation française.* Paris: Odile Jacob, 2018.

Debré, Robert. *L'Honneur de vivre.* Paris: Hermann, Editeurs des Sciences et des Arts, 1996.

D'Estienne d'Orves, Rose and Philippe, *Honoré d'Estienne d'Orves: Pionnier de la Résistance. Papiers, carnets et lettres,* Paris: Editions France-Empire, 1985.

Doulut, Alexandre; Klarsfeld, Serge, and Lebeau, Sandrine. *Les Rescapés juifs d'Auschwitz témoignent.* Paris: Les Fils et Filles des Déportés Juifs de France, Après l'Oubli, 2015.

Drogland, Joel. *Des maquis au Morvan au piège de la Gestapo: André Rondenay, Agent de la France Libre.* Paris: Vendémiaire, 2019.

Fette, Julie. *Exclusions. Practicing Prejudice in French Law and Medicine 1920–45.* Ithaca, NY: Cornell University Press, 2012.

Halioua, Bruno. *Blouses blanches et étoiles jaunes.* Paris: Editions Liana Levi, 2002.

Hautval, Adélaïde. *Médecine et Crimes Contre l'Humanité.* Paris: Actes Sud, 1991.

Lalieu, Olivier. *La Zone Grise? La Résistance française à Buchenwald.* Paris: La Grand Livre du Mois, 2005.

Leriche, René. *Souvenirs de ma vie morte.* Paris: Seuil, 1958.

Manhès, Frédéric-Henri. *Buchenwald: L'Organisation et L'Action Clandestine des Déportés Français 1944–1945.* Paris: FNDIRP (Fédération nationale des déportés et internés, résistants et patriotes), 1947.

Marin, René. *Un Enfant a vécu le massacre de Dun-les-Places (Juin 1944): Il Raconte.* Dun-les-Places, self-published, 2014.

Marrus, Michael R., and Robert O. Paxton. *Vichy France and the Jews.* New York: Basic Books, 1981.

Merle d'Aubigné, Robert. *Une Trace.* Paris: La Table Ronde, 1987.

Michelet, Edmond. *Rue de la Liberté. Dachau 1943–45.* Genève: Editions de Crémille, 1971.

Milliez, Paul. *Médecin de la liberté.* Paris: Editions du Seuil, 1982.

Monod, Claude. *La région D, rapport d'activité des maquis de Bourgogne-Franche-Comté.* Saint-Etienne-Vallée-Française: Aiou, 1993.

Monod, Robert. *Les Heures Décisives de la Libération de Paris (9–26 Août 1944)*. Paris: Editions Gilbert, 1947.

Nahum, Henri. *La Médecine française et les Juifs 1930–1945*. Paris: Editions L'Harmattan, 2006.

Odic, Charles-Jean. *'Stepchildren' of France*. Translated from the French by Henry Noble Hall, New York: Roy Publishers, 1945.

Orlowski, Dominique, dir. *Buchenwald, par ses témoins. Histoire et dictionnaire du camp et ses kommandos*. Paris, Belin, 2014.

Pasteur Vallery-Radot, Louis, *Mémoires d'un non-conformiste*. Paris: Plon, 1970.

Poznanski, Renée. *Les Juifs en France pendant la Seconde Guerre Mondiale*. Paris: Hachette, 1994.

Procès des Grand Criminels de Guerre devant le Tribunal Militaire International. Nuremberg: Tribunal Militaire International, 1946–49, Vol. VI.

Prochiantz, Alec. *Promenons-nous dans les bois*. Paris: Société des écrivains, 2011.

Prost, Antoine, dir. *La Résistance, une histoire sociale*. Paris: Editions de l'Atélier, 1997.

Richet, Charles; Richet, Jacqueline and Richet, Olivier. *Trois Bagnes*. Paris: J. Ferenczi et fils, 1945.

Richey, Paul. *Fighter Pilot. A Personal Record of the Campaign in France 1939–1940*. Stroud, Gloucestershire, UK: The History Press (reprint), 2016.

Roelke, Volker, Sascha Topp, and Etienne Lepicard, eds. *Silence, Scapegoats, Self-reflection: The Shadow of Nazi Medical Crimes on Medicine and Bioethics*. Göttingen, Germany: V&R Press, 2011.

Rousset, Jean. *Chez les Barbares*. Lyon: La Guillotière, 1946.

Un Secteur de la Résistance française. Livre blanc sur Buchenwald. Paris: Editions de la Résistance et de la déportation, 1955.

Vergez-Chaignon, Bénédicte. *Les Internes des hôpitaux de Paris 1802–1952*. Paris: Hachette, 2002.

Vial, Robert. *Histoire des Hôpitaux de Paris dans l'Occupation. Les Blouses blanches dans l'étau de Vichy et l'espoir de Londres*. Paris: L'Harmattan, 1999.

Vigreux, Marcel. *Les villages-martyrs de Bourgogne: 1944*. Saulieu: Association pour la recherche sur l'Occupation et la Résistance, 1994.

Wellsted, Ian. *SAS with the Maquis: In Action with the French Resistance*. Barnsley, South Yorkshire, UK: Frontline Books, 2016.

Wetterwald, François. *Vengeance: Histoire d'un corps franc*. Paris: Imprimérie J. Téqui, 1946.

Wieviorka, Annette, and Michel Laffitte. *A l'intérieur du Camp de Drancy*. Paris: Perrin, 2012.

Wormser, Olga, and Henri Michel. *Tragédies de la Déportation 1940–45. Témoignages des survivants des camps de concentration allemands*. Paris: Hachette, 1955.

INDEX